EVERY THREE HOURS

Janet Malcolm Hayles

EVERY THREE HOURS

A Mother's Story of Raising
a Child with Chronic Illnesses
from Car Seat to Career

Tarheel Shaw Writes

Some names and identifying details have been changed to protect the privacy of individuals.

Published by Tarheel Shaw Writes, Chapel Hill

GIRL FRIDAY PRODUCTIONS

Edited and designed by Girl Friday Productions
www.girlfridayproductions.com

Cover design: Emily Weigel
Project management: Reshma Kooner
Editorial production: Abi Pollokoff
Image credits: cover © Shutterstock/Nadiiiya

ISBN (paperback): 979-8-9865688-0-5
ISBN (e-book): 979-8-9865688-1-2

Library of Congress Control Number: 2022916908

To the parents of the nearly twenty million children with chronic illness and disabilities in the US: It's never going to be easy. You will walk with your child's condition the rest of your life; jump when the phone rings; celebrate the small victories. Can you help your child take those small steps forward to independence? It's worth everything you can give to it. And, along the way, you will find yourself changed—stronger, more introspective, and grateful for every positive moment.

CONTENTS

PART 3: WALKING FORWARD

PHOTOGRAPHS

ACKNOWLEDGMENTS

Martin Hayles: a wonderful father and support

Sammy Hayles: a man of incredible inner strength

Thomas Hayles: the older brother and mentor with unbelievable patience

Our family's "angels": Amy, Retha, Mrs. Mason, Mrs. Meeks, Dr. Rittler, Dr. Stanley, and Dr. Weinstein

INTRODUCTION

There are scores of books written about children with chronic medical conditions. Parents—mothers especially—recount their struggles with asthma, diabetes, cerebral palsy, sickle cell anemia, Down syndrome, cystic fibrosis, cancer, AIDS, and epilepsy.

However, this memoir is about two little-known medical conditions called glycogen storage disease type 1a and mast cell activation syndrome.

Why would I assume you would be interested in my experiences with my child's obscure medical conditions when you are exhausted and struggling as a mom of a child with the relatively common childhood condition of type 1 diabetes? Why would you be interested in what I have to say when we don't even know each other and our children's conditions are different? After all, you, Mom, are lying on the couch after a fifteen-hour day of attempting to manage your four-year-old's medical challenges. You're not sure you can face the blood-sugar ups and downs of tomorrow. You're not even sure you can scootch the Tinkertoys aside to get off the couch or put on clean socks.

But you know what? I am a mom just like you. We are the same mom, you and I. Millions of us are that mom. In total, we struggle with the fact that one-fourth of the children in our country today suffer from a chronic condition. *One-fourth.* As moms, we are not alone, and by sharing our experiences, we can help one another.

That is my reason for this memoir, the "so what" behind it, and why I am reliving much of the painful past. My reasons are twofold. First, I want to share with you my methodology for raising a chronically ill child—a child with two conditions that drug companies often ignore—to become an independent adult. Yet, it's amazing what a challenged child can do—step by step by step into adulthood. I don't profess to be an expert in children's chronic illnesses, but that's okay. I am simply a parent who worked as hard as she could with her child. My life has been full of bumbling, planning, researching, and crying for help. That may be where you are now. Stay tuned for some hope as well as hands-on techniques.

The second "so what" of this memoir is my personal journey and growth in raising a child with two chronic illnesses. Unfortunately, research today about chronically ill children and nurturing their independence isn't always helpful. Nearly all of the advice is framed in terms of parenting a five-year-old. For example, have him participate in household chores. Walk the dog. Be responsible for homework. But what if the "child" is nineteen years old and six foot two, and the independent act is one of traveling to India—eighty-two hundred miles away? It's a different scenario entirely. There's no road map for this. Here's the good news: *my* personal journey and growth can also become *your* personal journey, growth, and hope. What can we learn together, you and I?

My hope is that you will walk with me in this journey. You may find tears, and you may find smiles. Most importantly, you may find ways to help your child walk on, step by step by step, into a life of success, however that looks for him. Come with me. . . .

PART 1

DISCOVERY

1

In the Beginning

It was about 3:00 a.m. when the wailing began. This time, however, it was different. Plaintive and desperate.

I'm an experienced mom, I thought that night as I pulled myself upright in a pitch-dark haze. Just five years earlier, my first baby, Thomas, would fuss each night, and I would fly into his room for the three o'clock bottle. I would rock him, singing my favorite hymn. "Amazing grace! How sweet the sound that saved a wretch like me!" It was a peaceful time, nearly holy. No other sound except the rhythmic creak of my century-old oak rocking chair and soft slurps coming from Thomas. *This is the essence of life,* I would think, rocking back and forth. I remember the crescent moon outside the window, caught in the branches of our massive oak tree. After a nestle-down into the crib and a hefty burp, baby Thomas would move his thumb to his mouth and drift asleep.

It was now 1992: *this* time and *this* baby were different.

I had rolled out of bed each night when Sammy fussed, patting my husband Martin's inert body with an "I've got this." I was on maternity leave, while Martin put in at least sixty-five hours a week at a pharmaceutical company in Kansas City, our hometown. It was only fair. I normally fed Sammy once or twice a night.

Sammy was about four months old at the time, and I remembered how my baby books recommended that it was appropriate to let him "cry it out." That's what I had done with Tommy, so it was about time that Sammy should start following the plan. With my older son, I had perched on the stairs just feet from his room, hearing the wailing slowly drift to a shaky sniffle and then into silence in just a few minutes. All the while, I would bury my head in my hands and think, *This just seems wrong. Tommy may stop crying, but I am surely going to start.* But the baby books were right. Tommy began sleeping through the night after three nights of crying it out. While these episodes lasted only about five minutes, they seemed an endless torment to me. *How can this be good parenting?* I would think.

It was time for Sammy to follow the schedule too. I sat cross-legged in the hallway after his wails had reached me, but on this night, the cries sounded different. I rubbed my tired eyes in frustration as I thought of the words in my dog-eared baby book that explained the "cry-it-out method," saying babies would never learn to self-soothe if a parent always responded in the night. Okay, then. We were working on self-soothing here.

That night, Sammy's crying continued, building force. Five minutes. Ten minutes. What was this? Why was he not calming down? His well check with Dr. Willerton just two weeks ago had been uneventful. *What's going on, little man?*

That night, I finally grabbed the baby bottle, thinking, *To heck with the baby books. I'm feeding this child.* And so I did, night after night. Rocking in the old oak rocker, singing "Amazing Grace" and touching my face to Sammy's fuzzy-headed softness. The soft smells of Johnson's Baby Shampoo and Similac would drift up to me.

I was right to ignore the baby books. I would have killed my son if I had let him "cry it out."

2

The First of Many Doctors

About a week after I decided to throw the baby books out, I brought Sammy in to see Dr. Willerton, our family pediatrician. I was worried. I was feeding Sammy at least once in the middle of each night, as well as giving him six small feedings during the day. Sammy had been born with rounded baby cheeks, but he was getting a tummy too.

Dr. Willerton was a neighbor and had been Thomas's pediatrician. The doctor had weathered vaccinations, chicken pox, and midnight earaches with us. He had guided us through teething, fevers, splinters, and vomiting. Dr. Willerton, in short, was a beautiful combination of a wise Moses mixed with a cheerful Santa Claus. In thirty-five years of practice, he had seen it all.

I positioned Sammy on Dr. Willerton's examination table that day. The doctor always talked to Sammy, taking the baby's little hands in his own spotted ones. "And how are you today,

Mr. Sammy? Is your mother reading you some good stories? Have you picked out your university yet and declared a major?" Then Dr. Willerton would turn to me and ask, "Do you have any questions or concerns at this point?"

"Uh, yes. It seems like the last couple of days that Sammy is not urinating much. Can you take a look?"

Dr. Willerton carefully laid Sammy down on the exam table and peeled open the front of the Pampers. He carefully examined Sammy's little "man stuff." Being from Kansas, we never called things exactly what they were or said what we really thought. For example, buttocks were labeled "bunootskies," while a colonoscopy was called a "fooootamagoooot." If you owned a cool vest with fringe hanging off the bottom, well, that vest had "frabbers" on it. Don't ask me why.

Dr. Willerton thoughtfully examined Sammy, looking for lumps or malformations. Sammy responded by shooting forth a vigorous arc of urine right down the doctor's wool sweater, hitting three suede diamond patches on the front. Sammy's aim was spot-on. Dr. Willerton, always unflappable, looked at me with a grave face and crinkly blue eyes, joking, "Well, *that* part sure works!"

I wrestled with momentary mortification as the pediatrician carefully blotted yellow droplets from his pricey sweater. "Uh. I have another question." I described to him how Sammy had to be fed at least once every night and many times during the day. I was even putting a bit of baby cereal in the formula. Nothing seemed to curb Sammy's appetite.

Dr. Willerton carefully checked Sammy's temperature and gently probed the baby's glands, ears, eyes, and abdomen. He gently sat Mr. Cherub-Cheeks up, carefully running his finger along Sam's tummy and spine. Sam eyed the doctor, looking calmly at him with rounded blue eyes.

"Sammy is tilting his head to one side a bit. Do you see? It seems his neck muscles aren't strong enough to support his head. I think we should run some tests to rule out PKU, and we also may need to consider cerebral palsy. We'll also run routine lab work and a urinalysis."

"Wait. *What?*" The mention of cerebral palsy smacked my heart. I felt like my secure little world had just hit a brick wall. "And what's PKU?" This conversation just could not be happening.

Dr. Willerton explained calmly. "PKU is short for phenylketonuria. We can do a blood test to rule out this rare disorder. With PKU, children can't break down phenylalanine, an essential amino acid, so it builds up in their body, causing brain damage. The phenylalanine can also build up to dangerous levels if the baby has a lot of milk, cheese, or even grains.[1] Now, cerebral palsy is harder to diagnose. With cerebral palsy, a child can suffer from poor motor skills, as well as difficulties in eating and talking. We'll test for PKU and observe Sammy for a few months to note any signs of cerebral palsy. The lab work and urinalysis will check for infections, parasites, and so on."

Sammy had been having milk, cheese, and grains several times each day. Great. Purified cow's milk—whey protein. Baby cereal with rice flour, soy lecithin, and heaven knows what else. Had I unintentionally been harming my baby?

I didn't understand how Sammy could be sick. Martin and I were healthy: we ate broccoli by the bin full and worked out when we could. Our six-year-old Tommy was healthy, too, despite having run-ins with ear infections. Our parents were in great shape. Well, my dad had type 2 diabetes, but that was just because he was overweight and sedentary, wasn't it? This new situation didn't make sense to me. The cheerful blue-and-red pediatrician's room suddenly felt surreal and threatening.

"Let's just run these tests and see where we are." Dr.

---

1. "PKU," Mayo Clinic, last modified May 13, 2022, https://www.mayoclinic.org/diseases-conditions/phenylketonuria/symptoms-causes/syc-20376302#:~:text=Phenylketonuria%20(fen%2Dul%2Dkey,needed%20to%20break%20down%20phenylalanine.

Willerton was grave but calm, touching Sammy's fuzzy pink cheek with both a practiced doctor's hand and that of a grandpa. "Sometimes a baby's muscles just need more time to develop."

A little finger of fear wiggled in my gut. Cerebral palsy and PKU—these were serious things. They were not in my plan for life. But Dr. Willerton had *seemed* pretty calm, carefully closing Sam's chart with a suppressed sigh and patting the baby on the knee. As we left the pediatrician's, I attempted to quiet the fear inside me. On the way home, Sammy became busy shaking his stuffed toy monkey, Elmer, as he sat in his car seat. Mr. Monkey's eyes stared at me as I glanced in the rearview mirror of my old blue Volvo station wagon. The eyes seemed to mock me: *So, you think you've got life figured out?*

***

Two days later, I got Tommy fed and ready for school. It was the usual battle over clothes. Tommy, or Tee-Tee, as we called him, wanted to wear a Mutant Ninja Turtles tee shirt with electric-colored shorts. He selected bright blue socks, pulling them over his existing yellow socks. Apparently, socks were *always* itchy and annoying; "spicy," he called them. As Martin herded Tee into the car for school, the child looked like a circus clown ready to enter the ring at Barnum and Bailey. Tee didn't care. He was off for a big day in kindergarten. *We're making Oobleck today*—a white gooey clay from cornstarch—*and lunch is going to be cheese pizza. And Maryann hit me yesterday, and ick, she's a girl.*

Sammy and I spent four hours at Shawnee Mission Medical Center after Tee headed to school. We did blood work. Sammy howled, and we waited on stiff turquoise vinyl couches with blank walls staring at us. Minutes later, a young nurse fastened a plastic bag over Sammy's "little manhood" and popped on a new diaper. Even at four months, Sammy evidently knew things didn't feel right "down under," but collect urine we did. Sammy howled some more, and we waited again on *different* vinyl couches and stared at *new* blank walls. We did a mouth scrape for genetic testing. More howling and waiting and more vinyl couches with their crinkly cushions pressing unforgivingly into us. With Sammy still wet eyed from the morning's events, I carried him into the genetic counselor's office.

As Sammy slowly filled his diaper, I answered the counselor's questions. The room began to smell rather close.

Nope. I have no siblings. Well, I don't know. I guess my parents never got around to it. Mom told me once that kids were too expensive—but that I was loved, wanted, and needed.

My mom's still alive and eighty. I don't think she's ever been sick, except for a few colds. Even the cold viruses knew you didn't mess with my mom. Oh, Mom has one sister. Aunt Jan. She's five years younger. I don't think she's been sick much either, but she sure does have an attitude. Whooo. Don't mess with her.

Dad's seventy-eight. Well, he's pretty chunky and has type 2 diabetes, and he likes vanilla ice cream a lot. No, he's never been around toxic substances—unless you consider numbers kind of toxic. He's a finance professor. Cash flow and present value and all that stuff.

No, just one other son. Tommy is nearly six. He plays soccer and has a thing about scratchy socks. He's also stubborn, but he gets that from my husband, Martin. Yes, Tommy developed right on schedule—it was like the kid was reading the baby books. God knew he was dealing with parental rookies.

Martin? Oh. He's forty-one and I'm thirty-eight. My pregnancies? Both of them were easy, with normal deliveries. With Sammy, I was at my job all day—even went to the gym on my lunch hour. I was at home—about five thirty in the afternoon—when Sammy decided to arrive. I was knee-deep in making spaghetti, my favorite dish. The ob-gyn wouldn't even let me hang around and eat my simmering masterpiece. Something about how I was going to have the baby on the front porch of my home.

My grandpas? I never got to see either of them. I think my dad's dad died of pneumonia in 1928. The other grandpa had some allergies, but I don't know any more. His wife, my grandma, had to rotate different foods every three days for him. She would mix together certain herbs and light them in a little pot. Grandpa would lean over the vapors and inhale the smoke. I never did know how he died.

My grandmothers? Well, Mimi, my dad's mom, was a sweetie. A minister's wife who baked cinnamon rolls and played the organ in a funeral home in Hutchinson, Kansas. I think maybe she had diabetes, yet she loved to bake up a storm. My dad's favorite goodie when he was growing up was raisin pie. He talked about it all of my childhood. I mean, all of my childhood. In fact, in his search for the recipe, Dad wrote the cooking columnist Nan Wiley, published in the Kansas City Star *and syndicated over the country. Dad described his mother's decadent raisin pie and sent out an impassioned appeal. Within weeks, little old ladies all over the country sent Dad recipes for raisin pie. My mom made thirty raisin pies over the course of two years, and each one, according to my dad, "was pretty close, but not quite." Mom, who hated cooking, would sigh and set her perfectionist jaw with determination. She would make the perfect raisin pie.*

My other grandma? Well, she was fine and then got really lonesome and started smoking cigarettes. We'd find them all over her house when Mom and I would come to clean. Sometimes, Grandma Julia would get cross with me when I'd play in the birdbath in her backyard. Then, when I was about eight, she got really thin. I guess she was forgetting to eat. We moved her to a rest home in Emporia, Kansas, where I lived as a girl. The place smelled like urine and rubbing alcohol. Somehow, Grandma fell and broke a hip at the rest home. Mom and Dad took her to the hospital, and I never saw her alive again.

Martin's parents? Well, Mavis, his mom, is a vivacious, social redhead and a whiz at bunco and pokeno. You ought to see her—a cigarette dangling from her mouth while she plays the "Maple Leaf Rag" on the piano with dizzying speed. Grandpa Bob is a wiry little guy with a flat top, blazing blue eyes, and a huge smile with oversized dentures that remind me of Chiclets gum. Bob has had fried eggs, bacon, and Tang—the "drink of the astronauts"—every day for the past forty years. He seems pretty healthy, despite the cigarettes.

The genetic counselor took copious notes as I detailed the family history.

"Well, I'll be in touch with you in about two weeks. Before you leave, I'll need you to complete some blood work and a mouth scraping here at the hospital for further genetic analysis. When can Mr. Hayles come in? Once all the data is in, I'll send you a report and call you." The counselor stood up, signaling that the session was over. It was okay. Sammy's diaper was making our eyes water.

3

Enter the Redheaded Angel

The weeks flew by, with soccer practices for Tommy, mounds of dirty clothes, teacher conferences, and first-grade homework. "See, Tee? Here are two tennis balls, and I give you two more. Let's count them. How many?"

"Five!" Tee would always answer. Math was not his thing.

I had taught for five years but never could figure out the contrarian in Tee. If I said day, he said night. If I said yes, he said no. If I said that the sky was blue, he'd say, "Well, actually, it's azure."

Azure? How the heck had Tee learned that in first grade?

While Tee was in school, Sammy and I had a busy schedule. We'd stack blocks or read *Pat the Bunny* and *Goodnight Moon*. We'd look at black-and-white stylized images of faces. "Happy!" I'd say, pointing at one image. "Sad," gesturing to another. This was supposed to make Sammy brilliant. At six months of age, the baby would sit quietly for ten minutes at a time, intently listening to my stories. I'd never been around babies except for Tee. Unlike Sammy, Tee would listen to a story for two minutes and then crawl like a beetle to any shiny toy nearby. He'd swoosh magazines from the coffee table onto the floor in reckless piles. Tee loved to pound pegs into his toy workbench, pushing it aside in ten seconds to zoom over to Tinkertoys. Not so with Sammy, the contemplative Buddha.

I had another month before I had to head back to work. Martin and I decided that—at least for a while—we'd use a full-time caregiver in the home until Sammy could go to school. Martin worked long hours at a pharmaceutical company, and I was about to begin a new position with a telecommunications company. Life would turn into chaos soon.

I visited with one of my friends after church one Sunday. She was a pediatrician who was heading back to work part-time now that her son was in a full-day kindergarten. She told me about her sitter who was now available. Retha.

Angels come in a lot of sizes and shapes, and hair colors, some of which are red.

Retha was in her late thirties, like me, with a husband and two nearly grown children. A smallish woman with curly red hair and thick constellations of freckles, Retha hailed from the Missouri Ozarks. She'd tell me how she and Bobby, her husband, would go to "Wal-Marts" over the weekend, sometimes hitting a big sale on fishing equipment. She'd always manage to add an *s* on the end of every store's name. It was just her way. Retha also loved "Ventures," another discount store where she'd purchase Coke by the twelve-pack, supporting her two-cans-a-day habit.

Retha and I hit it off immediately. I loved her fifteen years of experience around babies. She was so calm and always knew what to do. Sure, I had my baby books and my two degrees, but I couldn't match Retha's firm but gentle ways. We worked together for four weeks, talking through the boys' schedules.

Retha and I were even on the same page with discipline. We both agreed that with Tee, Mr. Contrarian, consistency was vital. An occasional time-out for Tee in his little red chair could do wonders. Daily chores were a must, combined with positive feedback. Even Sammy, once he was able, would help put away the books and Tinkertoys typically strewn all over the family room.

Over the next few months, I got to know Retha's family. Bobby worked as a welder. Crystal and Scott were in high school—both with decent grades and part-time jobs. No one was a slacker in Retha's family. When Crystal got married to Robbie when she was eighteen, Tee was the ring bearer in the church wedding. That seven-year-old child was decked out in a white tux, a small black bow tie, and two pairs of socks, to avoid the "spiciness." He looked like Mr. GQ, and boy, did he know it. Double-sock layer and all—Tee marched down the aisle of Crystal's wedding with redheaded dignity. At the front of the church, he announced to the minister and congregation, "I got 'em! The rings! Here ya go!" The congregation burst into laughter, as Tee dropped the rings and they rolled down the chancel steps leading to the altar. Tee bolted for the rings, skidding to a halt on his knees right before the startled bridesmaids.

Within four weeks of working together, Retha and I became totally on the same child-rearing page. I was ready to launch into motherhood and career with child number two. Sammy was six months, and Tee was a six-year-old Tasmanian devil. Piece of cake, right?

4

On Becoming a Captain of Industry

I loved my lazy days at home with Sammy. Reading stories. Wandering over the hills in the bright blue baby jogger. Plinking the keys on Sammy's toy piano, singing Barney the dinosaur's favorite song, "I Love You." Lying in a patch of sun slanting across the family room carpet, with Sammy resting on my chest, his little breaths like soft angel puffs.

However, work was waiting.

I had been an English teacher for about five years before the boys were born. I taught seventh-grade English and later ran a reading laboratory for all the "sevies." It was rewarding work, especially when I saw a mental light switch on for my kids. When little Jason went from a third-grade reading level to the sixth in four months, it was the best. When John could contain his hyperactivity and tackle his fifteen spelling words, it was the best. He would allow me to place a gentle, encouraging hand on his shoulder—the only kind touch he would get during the week from anyone.

With my sevies, we'd do newspaper units, interviewing each other and creating eye-popping crime stories for the *Smith-Hale Daily.* Other weeks, the kids would create decorated cereal boxes to illustrate a book they had read. The front would be a picture representing the plot; the back, the story; the sides, characterization; and the bottom, setting. However, my favorite activity was teaching the kids how to write complete sentences. This simple skill would get them through high school English, I hoped.

A subject and a verb equal a complete sentence, right? Action verbs were no problem for the kids. "Throw." Throw a spit wad. "Run." Run from the teacher after you throw the spit wad. "Talk." Talk in class whenever possible. But then I had to teach "helping verbs." The kids could *not* get this idea. How can you "is"? How could they learn to recognize all twenty-three of these strange words? Why in the heck would they ever need these words? I got an idea in the middle of the night my first month of teaching: "Miss Butcher's Wild and Crazy Verbs."

"Am, is, are, was, were, being, been, be, have, has, had, do, does, did, will, would, shall, should, may, might, must, can, could!" On day one of this exercise, we would stand up in class, shouting out our list of helping verbs. "And what are these for?" I would ask the class, like a cheerleader shaking her Smith-Hale pom-poms. "To help with complete sentences," they would shout back. "Louder and again!" I would announce. "Am, is, are, was, were . . ." "Louder!" I'd say. "And what do these go with?" I'd question. "Action verbs," the kids would scream back, delighted that they had a fun, wild English teacher. We performed this frenzy of verbs daily for three weeks. At the end of it, the kids knew their helping verbs—boy howdy. The only mishap occurred one day when the principal made a surprise visit to our classroom. He had heard the ruckus echoing down the hall. "Am, is, are, was, were . . . ," we all shouted, the walls vibrating. The principal's eyes bugged out a bit as he hastily exited the classroom and closed the door. "Uh, verbs!" I cried out as he made a discreet exit. "Helping verbs!"

Years later, I ran into David, one of my third periods. "Am, is, are, was, were, being, been, be . . . ," he recited to me as he hung on a ladder, pulling cabling through ceiling tiles at Tee's school. David had become a successful electrician. "Mrs. Butcher, you taught me a lot about English. I feel like I learned to write good."

I was *so* happy. "Learning to write good" *was* good.

***

While I was dodging spitballs at the middle school and breaking up fights in the hallway, Martin was jetting off to New York City or having business dinners at the Hyatt in Kansas City. He was writing up white papers on Financial Accounting Standards Board (FASB) rulings and meeting with vice presidents. I felt my teaching simply paled by comparison. Plus, within four years, I was getting burnt out from teaching helping verbs and stopping flying pizza in the cafeteria. Additionally, the introvert in me wanted to crawl under a rock. Thirty sets of eyes looking at me at eight o'clock every morning? No way. The angst of repetition and being "on" seven hours a day—every day—wore me down.

So, during my five years of teaching, the "captain of industry" ambition started to rise in me. Why should Martin have a cool job, and not me? This new goal took seed and grew before I had even thought about having children. It was back in the days when I had energy and could keep my clothes clean for an hour and could get three complete sentences out at home. What would have happened if I had had a child with a "problem" while being a captain of industry? I never even considered the possibility.

I've never let details like education or work experience stand in my way. I had the goal in mind. So, while I was still teaching, I took the Graduate Management Aptitude Test (GMAT). The results: my verbal and communication skills were high. The math scores were embarrassingly low. "That 'new math' in fourth grade did me in," I ranted to Martin. "Those Venn diagrams—that's what did it. Who cares about union and intersection?" The truth is, I had cried in fourth grade over long division and could never understand the dreaded "story problem."

I began applying for a supervisory position with every midsized company in Kansas City. I interviewed. I role-played. I cranked out résumés. I called contacts. I touched base. I spit shined my shoes and put on my best suit—actually, my only suit.

Nothing. Every letter came back to me, stating, "While we appreciate your strong educational background and teaching experience, your skill sets are not a match for the position we are trying to fill." In other words, I discovered that two English degrees and a quarter would buy me a cup of coffee. It was depressing. I needed someone—anyone—to give me a chance.

In the midst of the job application bloodbath, I applied for the MBA program at Rockhurst University in Kansas City. After all, Martin and I were two cool "young urban professionals"—yep—the dreaded yuppies. Kids? Why on earth would I do that?

Rockhurst was known in the area to have a strong accounting and finance program, one in which I could work full-time and go to class two nights a week. We were told to expect eight to ten hours of homework on top of the coursework per week. Thirty-six graduate classes plus fourteen hours of prerequisites for those of us who were liberal arts people. Easy peasy, right? At any rate, the gods were with me. The school must have looked at my university transcripts and skimmed over the puny GMAT math score. I got into the MBA program.

Not only were the graduate gods with me that week, but the job gods were also. I talked to a friend one day in the checkout line at Pak 'N Save. Her sister's aunt's neighbor was leaving her position as a legal secretary at United Telecommunications, the parent company for fourteen telephone companies around the country.

Hmmmm. Legal secretary. Get my foot in the door. Why not? I could type; I could quickly learn the Gregg shorthand system at the local community college. Sure, why not?

I got the job. I arrived on day one in my beige suit. I began hammering out legal contracts on my IBM Selectric with Wite Out tape perched nearby, praying that I could avoid typos as I peered at my boss's scrawling longhand that filled page after page of legal tablets. What were "access charges"? Would I know an analog signal if it flowed by me? I simply didn't know the telecommunications terminology. I hammered out those contracts. Page after page. Rewrite after rewrite. As the months clicked by, I was knee-deep in legal lingo and had completed my first two graduate prerequisite classes.

Within eighteen months, I had completed six courses and received a promotion from legal secretary to accountant in general accounting. Even though I was Miss Puny Math Score, I loved accounting and understood it. It was logical and balanced. Plus, it didn't talk back to me like my sevies had. If I stuck ten dollars on the debit side of a ledger, I had to do the same on the credit side. The tick-and-tie control freak inside of me loved the symmetry—it was nearly as satisfying as organizing my Little Golden books as a child. *Beauty and the Beast, Cinderella,* and then *Dumbo*, right? So, it was little wonder that I decided to go for an undergrad accounting degree while I was in school at Rockhurst. What was another twenty hours? I plowed through Beginning Accounting I and II and into Intermediate Accounting I and II, the two "killer requisites" of an accounting degree. Advanced Accounting. Cost Accounting. Managerial Accounting. Federal Tax. Budgeting. My debits and credits knew no end.

The months continued to fly by as I completed course after course. At work, I moved into Consolidation Accounting, Information Technology, and finally, Employee Benefits. It was all challenging and *so fun*. I would take a bank statement and wrestle with the fact that the company records had a totally different starting balance than the bank had. How could that *even happen*? I had to get this to agree—no Unlocated Difference (ULD) for this lady. In Information Technology, my boss, Ken, and I would crack open new computers and load software. We would teach employees about the horrors of typing in "Format C." We would travel to various companies to investigate new types of accounting consolidation software. I would fend off the Ernst & Young year-end auditors with my tidy and meticulous data schedules. I was like my lab, Georgie, who loved to wriggle on her back in the backyard, kicking her feet up in sheer joy. In short, I loved each area of United Telecommunications and became accustomed to jumping into a new position every two years or so. And I eventually got out of graduate school, nine months pregnant with Tee. I had been at Rockhurst so long—for six years—I halfway expected the university to name a building after me.

I was so naive at age thirty-two. I had left a teaching career that would have worked well with having a family. Martin and I had gotten the baby bug when I turned thirty-one, and presto chango, along came Tee. I never even thought how I would manage a corporate career and a child.

5

Home on the Range

Time whipped by. Tee was such a delight as a child, despite his spicy socks issue. Why not have another? Sure! Bingo! Enter Sammy.

I remember when Sammy turned eight months old. The days and months had flown by in a pattern—as much of a pattern as you can have with children.

I'd get home each day promptly at six o'clock, because Retha had a family to get home to, also. My heels flung by the front door with a clatter. The briefcase dumped on the stairs down to the family room with a thud. A hug for Tee-Tee. A kiss for Sammy. A debriefing with Retha. Five more minutes of visiting with the kids and then I'd head straight to the kitchen, stripping off my suit jacket, ready to cook. Maybe spaghetti and meatballs. A savory roast steaming in the Crock-Pot. Beef stew reheating after the weekend marathon of cooking. Martin usually got home at six thirty, and we all ate as a family soon after. Death, taxes, and children's hunger would never wait.

***

Sammy's tests for PKU had come back normal, as did his blood work. He showed no overt signs of cystic fibrosis. Although Sam wasn't extremely active like Tee, I inwardly relaxed; the fear in my gut transferred to work instead.

I had learned just before my second maternity leave that I was to be promoted as senior manager of employee benefit administration and accounting. It was a mouthful of a title, but little did I know what I was walking into.

Our small group at work had deferred-compensation plans to manage, as well as a below-market stock purchase plan, a Tax Reduction Act Stock Ownership Plan (TRASOP), and an old Employee Stock Ownership Plan (ESOP), to boot. I learned quickly that no documentation existed at all on these plans—just reams of employee distribution printouts. I *did* know from my classes at Rockhurst that any missed distributions to employees and executives would trigger massive tax liabilities for United Telecom. It would also trigger massive anger from any employees who didn't get their distributions or didn't get to enroll in a stock plan. Additionally, the gentleman who was relieved of running these plans when I took over was none too pleased. All I could get out of him was that each program ran on COBOL. "But," he'd tell me, "for *these* seven individuals, the program has a glitch. You need to update these seven Excel spreadsheets every quarter for these individuals." *Great,* I thought. *What a big opportunity for error here.* We might as well have used hamsters inside a spinning cage to power the benefit plans. What made matters worse: my new boss was the pension trust officer. His full-time accountability was making sure the company's pension was fully funded, so that company retirees got a pension plan and *kept* a pension plan. For administering the benefit plans—my boss relied on me. Adding to this poisonous mess was the fact that one of the department members was angry at me. She had wanted my job and was *sure* she had deserved it.

6

Missed Signals

To this day, I am haunted by the fact that I may not have been on top of Sammy's growing medical issues. I cooked for my boys, read stories, played Legos. It wasn't enough.

After one particularly grueling workday, I did my usual toss of shoes and briefcase on my scramble down the stairs into the family room. It was my ritual to hug the boys and visit with Retha every time I got home. In her calm manner, Retha was instructing the boys to clean up their toys, part of her daily routine with the kids. Tee made pot shots of Legos into his red toy bin, while Sammy merely scootched *Goodnight Moon* around the carpet.

Retha quietly got me over into a corner of the kitchen. "Um. I think Sammy's tummy is too large," stated Retha. "It doesn't look quite normal."

What? Huh? Sammy was only the second baby I'd been around in my life. True, he had chubby legs and round cheeks.

He used to create quite a stir in Pak 'N Save as the personification of the Gerber baby, with his huge blue eyes and blond curls. Later, as I changed Sammy's diaper, I looked at his tummy. Well, it did look a bit big, compared to Tee's at that age. However, Tee had always been skinny and active. I made a mental note to book an appointment with Dr. Willerton. Life had hummed along for several months, and, outside of frequent feedings, I didn't notice anything alarming about Sammy.

***

In August 1993, at the baby's twenty-month mark, we saw Dr. Willerton.

"Look at his tummy." I gestured to the pediatrician. "Does this look too big?" Retha's recent words echoed in my head.

Dr. Willerton carefully touched and manipulated Sammy's stomach, holding two fingers against the right side of the tummy and tapping against them with the other hand, moving the fingers of the bottom hand, and tapping again. His head was bent, listening.

"Uh, well." The mom in me tried not to sound ignorant as I phrased my question to the pediatrician. I questioned Dr. Willerton: "Should Sammy be getting ready to walk now? He crawls but doesn't even try to pull himself up." I had been working with Sammy for several weeks now, standing him up and gently holding onto his arms. Sam would simply crumple back into a sitting position. Anxiety was taking hold of me, seeping around my heart, my gut, my mind.

"Mr. Sammy, what's going on with you?" Dr. Willerton asked gently as he examined feet, arms, tummy, ears, eyes, mouth, and head posture.

The pediatrician stood quietly for a moment, flipping through Sammy's medical records and tapping his cheek.

"Let's schedule an ultrasound of Sammy's abdomen in the next two or three weeks. I also want you to begin taking Sammy to Childwise Physical Therapy. We need to see if we can strengthen those legs. Let's also get an appointment with Dr. Grace Somer. She's a cognitive assessment specialist."

Whoa. Something scary was happening here. This was not part of my plan. More anxiety seeping in.

The next few weeks were a flurry of activity despite my fears. At work, I dug into benefit plans, examining printout after printout, analyzing how the numbers were calculated. I met with our legal department to find out plan parameters. I met with programming so we could move from hamster-and-wheel processing to a more effective programming language. I met with department members to discuss their goals and training desires. I wrote up quarterly personnel reviews. I felt as though I were slowly crawling into a place of light and of understanding my position. It was exhilarating; I was using my brain to the fullest. But maybe . . . maybe . . . I wasn't mindfully present at home.

Three times a week, I'd meet Retha nearby when she was picking up Tee from school. I'd transfer Sammy from her car seat to mine, and we'd head out to Childwise PT.

Amanda was a pediatric physical therapist at Childwise. She had brown hair pulled into a perky ponytail. Her nursing uniforms were happy: dancing bunnies or prancing ponies. I loved Amanda's calmness—the way her hazel eyes truly examined Sammy.

I told Amanda that Sammy was not bearing much weight on his legs at twenty months. Nor had he attempted to pull himself up or take those few halting steps that I longed to see. In essence, Sammy seemed perfectly content to sit as I would read story after story to him.

At each PT session, I would sit by Amanda and observe her techniques, because I would have homework from these sessions. Amanda would carefully lift Sammy onto a small stool, placing his bare feet on the floor. "Look!" she'd exclaim, pointing to Barney the dinosaur on the floor close by. Sammy was supposed to get up and grab Barney and then sit back on the stool. Sammy looked at Barney—his favorite television character—but didn't move.

Amanda, Sammy, and I also practiced "cruising." We'd head to the nearby couch with a teddy bear set at one end. Amanda would place Sammy at one end of the couch, his hands positioned on the cushions. "Let's go get that teddy bear!" she'd say. Amanda and I would cruise down the length of the couch, our hands patting the cushions with happy slaps, our knees pressing into the red and blue blocks of carpeting. I would look at Sammy expectantly: "Come on, buddy!" Sammy would look at me and simply slide into a sitting position.

Amanda and I would hold Sammy gently by his upper arms and move one shoulder forward slightly, then the other. This motion was supposed to encourage Sammy's lower body to follow suit and move the legs. One leg would come forward. Then—plop—down Sammy would go, his blue eyes blinking as if to say, *I'm done here.*

Sammy's favorite PT activity was bicycling. Amanda would lay him on his back and "pedal" his legs, carefully extending and contracting the muscles. Sam would beam and smile. "Mo!" More.

Sammy and I would practice these PT moves each evening after dinner. "Come on, Tee; help us," I'd encourage. Soon, Martin, Tee, and I would be cruising down the family room couch. Slap slap slap. Sam would stand holding onto the end of the couch and look at us, implying, *You're all kind of acting strange.* Our favorite family activity, however, was the bicycling. We'd all be on our backs, pedaling in the air, belting out Barney the dinosaur's song. We looked like a family of struggling June bugs.

One night, Martin was in a work meeting, so the remaining Team Hayles did PT. I ran upstairs for a minute to start the daily laundry load. "Tee—would you bicycle with Sammy while I throw in the laundry?" Tee was the typical, responsible older brother, but his caregiving didn't always go as I planned. "Sure, Mom," he replied. I came downstairs within a minute or two, and what did I see? Sammy was wrapped in his baby blanket—his dee dee—a tattered piece of flannelly love. Tee had secured Sammy wonton style in the dee dee, slowly dragging him all over the family room carpet, crying, "Booster jets! Booster jets!" I rushed into the family room, alarmed by the sound of "booster jets" in my house. However, Sammy was laughing with delight during his dee dee ride. Tee pulled him slowly, around and around the family room, into the kitchen, and back out, with our lab, Georgie, trotting behind in excitement. Slowly, Sammy's wonton wrap came loose, and the child quickly rolled once, twice, six times, coming to a stop two inches from the family room wall. "Mo mo!" he shrieked. "Mo mo dee dee ride."

Two weeks after the PT marathons began, I took Sammy to Dr. Grace Somer, a physician specializing in cognitive assessment. As each week passed by, I was becoming more concerned by Sammy's lack of physical movement. Sometimes, he seemed like a floppy rag doll. He could sit on the carpet, heels of the feet touching, knees spread open wide to the floor. The child had learned to crawl to his toys, but nothing more. However, I was pretty sure his brain was working just fine. Words were beginning to flow out faster and faster. "Want a dee dee ride," Sammy would say, or "Have some cheese crackers." One day, as I thumped down the stairs after work, Retha met me on the landing, slightly breathless.

"Sammy just crawled up to me and said, 'Retha, I'm uncomfortable. I think I need a Tylenol.'"

What had been simmering in this child's brain? "Uncomfortable? Tylenol?" Really?

At the two-hour session with Dr. Somer, the specialist performed a variety of exercises to determine whether Sammy's brain was developmentally sound. Her room was quiet, peaceful, filled with bright, enticing puzzles. I was a bit envious of Sam. This looked like fun.

"What will you be evaluating in Sammy?" I asked Dr. Somer.

"I'm going to observe Sammy's verbal skills, verbal reasoning, novel-problem-solving, new task learning, and decision-making speed," the specialist replied, flipping through Sam's medical records on a clipboard. I told Dr. Somer about Sammy's unusual ability to sit and listen to stories—now, for up to fifteen minutes at a time. I told her about the incident Retha reported when Sammy had gushed forth two complete sentences.

"Interesting," she commented, scribbling away on her pad and then pausing to watch Sammy. Dr. Somer then lowered herself behind a low Plexiglas wall with a red ball. Sammy was on the other side.

"Sammy. Look at this ball! Can you get it?" Dr. Somer waved the red ball enticingly.

The child immediately reached around the wall and took the ball. He bounced it away, as if to say, *Now whatcha got?*

"What did that just show you?" I asked Dr. Somer.

"In slower cognitive development, the child won't realize that he can reach around the wall. He'll try to reach directly to the ball. He wouldn't understand that the clear Plexiglas is blocking his grasp."

"Well, what will all these other puzzles and games tell you?" I prodded Dr. Somer with more questions. I was thinking, *Is Sammy pretty smart?*

"I'm observing to see if Sammy might have any intellectual

disabilities or processing problems that might impact the brain-to-body movement. Has he had any brain injuries?"

Outside of the wild dee dee escapade a few days ago, Sammy had had no incidents. I did tell Dr. Somer about his need for frequent feedings and muscle weakness and floppiness.

A week later, I received a report in the mail from Dr. Somer. She was pleased to inform us that Sammy had "advanced cognitive ability." So why couldn't the child walk? Something was wrong with my baby.

7

What Was Wrong with Sammy?

When Sammy was twenty months old, Martin and I brought him in for the ultrasound of his abdomen at Shawnee Mission Medical Center. Sammy had continued to spout words at a breathtaking rate. However, he was still not walking, choosing instead to crawl after Georgie. The wiggle of fear in my gut had been growing stronger.

I still remember him. James, the technician in the ultrasound room, looked like a Kansas City Chiefs defensive end. Big burly arms coming out of his technician's white coat. Crinkly brown eyes that radiated kindness. A cap of curly black hair.

James and Martin placed Sammy on his back on the white bed, and the child immediately tensed. The technician tickled Sammy's tummy and said, "Now, Mr. Sammy, we're going to put this gel on your tummy, and then I'm going to roll this fairy wand around and around on your belly to take a look inside your tummy. It's magic." He let Sammy touch the special wand. James placed a dollop of the warmed ultrasound gel on Sammy's belly and began to slowly roll the fairy wand, first on one portion of the stomach and then the next. He would pause, studying the ultrasound screen carefully. "I'm looking at the gallbladder now." He would measure the organ on the screen, capture an image, and type in numbers. "I'm also looking at the liver, spleen, and pancreas. I'll be also viewing the inferior vena cava and aorta." Red and white surges of light appeared on the ultrasound screen, pulse-like, unnervingly psychedelic.

Mid-ultrasound, Sam protested, "No sauce! No sauce!" against the gooey ultrasound gel and the gentle wand circling on his tummy. He wound himself up into a soppy crying fit. The technician, unperturbed, captured more images and measured each organ. "It's okay, Mr. Sammy. We're almost done." I held the child's hand and stroked his baby curls with one finger. "When we get home, we'll read *Goodnight Moon*," I encouraged. "We'll go to the park with Tee tomorrow."

The ultrasound session was over. Martin hugged Sammy as I gathered my purse and the diaper bag. I'm not sure who was the more dewy-eyed from the ordeal. Two sets of teary blue eyes looked at me. "Okay, buddy?" The technician did a quick tickle under Sammy's chin.

Two days later, the radiologist had the ultrasound report faxed to Dr. Willerton. The pediatrician called me that afternoon at work.

"Janet, I've just looked at this report. Sammy has an enlarged liver."

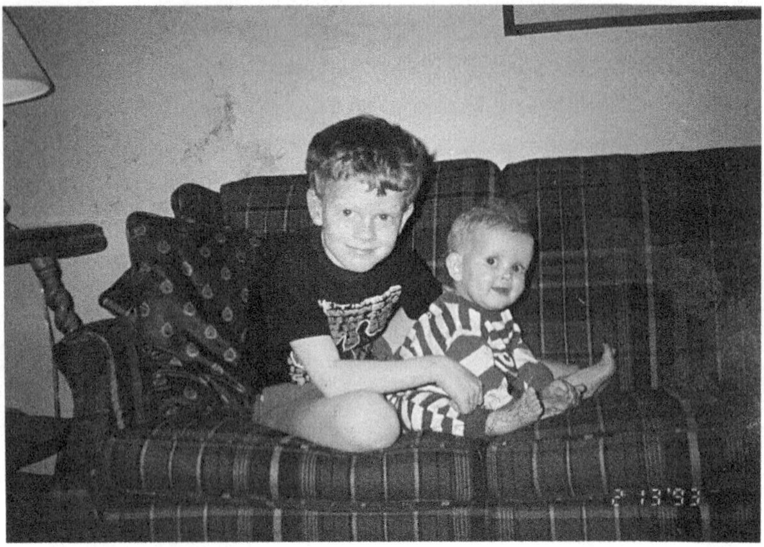

Tee and Sammy, ages six and one

8

Now What Do We Do?

I don't remember the rest of the conversation with Dr. Willerton. Something about "Please call me any time" and "Bring Sammy in tomorrow at Shawnee Mission Medical Center for additional blood work and a CAT scan."

Something was wrong. Really wrong with my baby.

I went into my boss's office and told Bill what had just happened. I had to go home. I felt sick—that kind of heartsick feeling when you see a bad car accident. I had to hold Sammy—to feel, somehow, that this was just a nightmarish dream. Not my baby. Not this.

I got home somehow, not remembering the streets I took. I tried to think through my fear. I had taken two measly science courses in college. I was clueless about medical issues. I knew that the liver was in the abdomen—on the side, perhaps? All I could think of was hepatitis C, cirrhosis of the liver,

liver cancer. Did they enlarge the liver? All of the conditions sounded terrible and deadly.

When I got home, I sneaked Retha over into a corner of the kitchen and told her the frightening report on Sammy's enlarged liver.

"I wonder if that's what's making his tummy so large?" Retha began to tear up, her freckled hand up to her mouth to suppress a cry. She and I hugged in a desperate mom-to-mom silent plea for help. Retha hurried up the stairs so Sammy and Tee wouldn't see while I blinked and wiped my eyes on a rumpled dish towel. I remember wandering into the family room, seeing the two boys playing Legos in all their innocence. In their worlds, nothing was wrong. Tee had on a shiny tinfoil crown from school labeled "Super Reader." Sammy shoved his Cheez-Its aside as he crawled to me, his cherub cheeks popping a grin. We three sat in the slanted late-afternoon sunshine in our family room, racing Lego fire trucks and putting together large wooden puzzles. In the sickness of my heart, I thought, *How many times have I sat here with my boys, just taking this peacefulness, this grace of children, all for granted?*

As soon as I heard the click-click of Martin's dress shoes in the upstairs hallway, I bolted up to him. I needed to share my fear with someone special—someone wise and calm like Martin. Martin had a business and law background, with an enduring love of Bible study. In short, Martin was a beautiful combination of brains, spirituality, and just plain horse sense.

"The radiologist's report came back today. Dr. Willerton called me and said that Sammy's liver is enlarged." I grabbed Martin's arm for support, as we both sat at the top of the stairs. Martin would know what to do here. He always knew what to do.

I still remember Martin's face turning slightly gray at that moment. I'm not sure how we got through the evening. We fixed dinner, supervised bath time, and read stories to the kids just like always, because we had to. Somehow, there was a bit of comfort in the routine. *Maybe life is really normal, and the ultrasound was a fluke.* At eight thirty, Martin took Sammy for tuck-in while Tee and I headed to his room. I was in no mood to be a disciplinarian that night, so I let Tee ride the swinging wooden wolf that Grandpa Bob had made for him. It hung on sturdy ropes from the rafters in his room. Back and forth Tee raced, nearly hitting each wall and crying out, "Booster jets! Booster jets!" Then, with Tee pj'd up and tucked under his Ninja Turtle sheets, we wrapped up our bedtime ritual. I raised my arms and hands apart, as if I were measuring the field goals at the Chiefs' football stadium.

"I love you this much!" I'd exclaim, with my arms spread out.

"How much?" Tee would reply, his blue eyes just daring me.

"*This* much!" My arms would widen.

"Howwwwwww much?" Tee's toothy smile would widen.

"*Thiiiiiiiiiiis* much!" My arms would spread as far as they could go.

It was beautiful. For just a moment, I forgot the sickness in my heart as I kissed Tee's freckled nose.

***

Later that night, Martin and I sat with glasses of wine and a pad of paper, trying to think of where we could go for help. Dr. Willerton had sensed something was wrong with Sammy for months, but all the test results had come back marked "normal" until the ultrasound. "Perhaps see Dr. Atherton. He's a hepatologist at Shawnee Mission Medical Center," our kindly pediatrician had suggested. "He helps patients manage disorders of the liver, the gallbladder, and the pancreas." Dr. Willerton was a good thirty-five years out of medical school. He knew *something* was wrong, but what?

Should we go to other specialists also? Martin worked for a large pharmaceutical company, but he was in purchasing. Everyone in our extended family was either a teacher or in business. No doctors. No science backgrounds. No clue.

How many other parents were sitting somewhere that same evening, struggling with frightening medical test results? Thousands. And, like us, they sat and brainstormed, trying to think of something—anything—that could begin to help their child.

"What about Carol Morrison at church?" my husband finally suggested. "She's a pediatrician. . . . Only been out of school about seven years. Let's call her tomorrow." The two of us headed to bed, sleeping poorly. A black mist of fear hovered over us.

The next morning, Martin headed out the door to take Tee to school while I took a personal day to regroup and to push my sick fear into a safe little box. As soon as the clock hit eight thirty, I called Carol. She and I often talked after church over coffee and donuts in the narthex. Ours was a small church of eighty parishioners—everyone knew everyone. We all pitched in to clean the church and haul away the trash each Saturday. When the minister's son picked his nose during the children's sermon, everyone grinned. When our son Thomas goosed a kid with a palm frond on Palm Sunday, everyone grinned. There were no secrets.

I described to Carol what the radiologist's report had said. "Come on over," Carol said. Sitting at her kitchen table with coffee minutes later, I held the squirming Sammy in my arms. Carol gently felt his tummy.

"One of my professors in school was Dr. Marris, head of genetics at Children's Mercy Hospital in downtown Kansas City. I'd go see him. He's very knowledgeable about genetic issues, and I think he could help you get a handle on this."

Genetic issues? My child? No one in our family had had

any weird medical issues that I knew of. People died from broken hips or diabetes or just old age. Plus, I had undergone an amniocentesis with both pregnancies. Apparently, with my first pregnancy at age thirty-two, I was "mature" and therefore a risk. I was thirty-eight and "very mature" when Sammy was born in 1992. I had decided to receive the slightly risky test procedure because my obstetrician had informed me that an amniocentesis would detect chromosome abnormalities, neural-tube defects, and genetic disorders, such as Down syndrome or cystic fibrosis. *Well,* I had thought, *it is* not *part of my plan to have a child with a "problem." Martin and I are too healthy, and that just won't happen.* And I was quickly reassured that life would be okay as results from each amniocentesis came back labeled "within normal range." I was ready to have that second child, a healthy baby, according to my tidy little schedule.

9

A Glimmer of Insight

On Monday morning after the visit with Carol, I was on the telephone to Children's Mercy Hospital. Incredibly, I got an appointment with Dr. Marris for the following week. A small beam of hope pushed at the sick feeling that had been in my stomach since I had learned of Sammy's enlarged liver.

After our thirty-minute uneventful trek into Children's Mercy, we wound up and up the layers of parking of the hospital. Sammy and I walked down hallways and more hallways, to elevators and more elevators, and into the genetics department.

The genetics waiting room was purposefully cheerful. Sammy and I checked in and headed over to a large play wall with moving plastic gears and blue spinning wheels. The couches and chairs in the large room were happy reds, yellows, and blues. Framed pictures of children's art decorated each wall. The room seemed to say, *We know you're here with a sick child. We're going to pretend everything is pleasant.* I looked around. Sammy had made a new friend, a freckled girl who appeared to be about three or four.

"See? Spin this dial," Sam explained to the new friend.

"Da," the child stated. She tried to push the dial but couldn't get her hand to do it. "Da."

By this time, Sammy had crawled over to a colorful tic-tac-toe mat, pushing each square for a satisfying "ding." His friend was still at the dial, staring at it. I looked around. Parents sat here and there in the waiting room, holding babies with nasogastric tubes or parking strollers with loaded diaper bags. One small boy was wheeled out of the appointment room in his miniature wheelchair, an IV in his arm and a mask over his face. Another child walked by with one healthy arm, but the other one was just a stub. I was taken aback. I had never seen so many children with physical challenges in one place. Sammy and I didn't belong in this place with *sick* children, did we? I mean, these kids were really, really sick. Was Sammy?

"Mrs. Hayles and Sammy?" It was time for our appointment.

I looked at Dr. Marris expectantly as we entered his office, because he was my hope and my only hope for explaining and "fixing" this liver nightmare. I remember his crisp shirt and pinstripe tie. Definitely Brooks Brothers. The doctor's gray eyes peered at me from behind tortoiseshell glasses. Knowledgeable eyes, but cold eyes.

"Sammy's over twenty months now and still not walking," I told Dr. Marris. "He'll try to pull up to walk but just falls down. I feed him about seven times a day because he acts hungry. And here's the radiology report."

Dr. Marris took copious notes, flipped through the radiology report, and then carried Sammy over to his examination table. Gentle hands palpated the child's tummy here and there. Capable hands sat Sammy up as the geneticist observed the cute little tilting head. Knowledgeable hands probed Sammy's range of motion with his legs. They were pliable and floppy.

I wriggled a bit on the office chair. My hopes and my fears fought, making my heart thump. Sammy looked so cute and vulnerable on Dr. Marris's exam table—huge blue eyes taking in everything around him.

After minutes ticked by, Dr. Marris handed Sammy to me and sat in his office chair.

"Well," he said, clearing his throat. *Well, what?* My gut continued to churn.

"Based on my exam and the test results here, I believe Sammy has a form of glycogen storage disease."

I interrupted Dr. Marris. "What? Wait a minute. Wait a minute. I've never heard of this. Why didn't Dr. Willerton diagnose this? What is this glycogen thing?" In my state of panic, sentences just flew out of me.

Dr. Marris didn't say anything but leaned forward in his chair, staring me into quietness.

"Based on what I'm seeing, I think Sammy has a *less* severe form of glycogen storage disease. There are about sixteen kinds that have been discovered so far. If I had to take a guess, I'd say he has GSD type IIIa, which you'll sometimes hear referred to as Forbes disease. We won't know for sure what kind of GSD Sammy has until we perform a needle biopsy of his liver and take some tissue samples." The words "needle biopsy" circled ominously in my brain. What was glycogen? Was a needle biopsy dangerous? I kissed the top of Sammy's head, needing comfort and grounding. Sammy was so innocent, so vulnerable.

"It's rare, one occurrence per one hundred thousand babies born. Many doctors have only read a page or two about the condition—usually in medical school. Can you feel his large liver, here? It's storing excessive glycogen. And his round cheeks are storing adipose tissue."

"Um," I said, as though my intelligence had all been sucked away in the fluorescent-lit room. "My degrees are in English and finance. I'm really lost here. Will Sammy be okay? Do you think he will ever be able to walk?" Nightmares began to circle me.

Dr. Marris looked a bit irritated but continued. "Patients with GSD will have a certain enzyme in the liver that's either missing or mutated. It's a recessive genetic disorder that both you and your husband have. When you conceived, Sammy had a one-in-four chance of getting GSD."

"So . . . so . . . so . . ." I was babbling. I had to talk fast before Dr. Marris would whisk out of the room and on to other "interesting" genetic mysteries.

"When you and I eat a meal," he said, "our bodies get glucose from food and convert it into *glycogen*, which is stored in the liver for future use. Our bodies need glucose all the time. It appears that Sammy's liver cannot convert much, if any, glycogen back into glucose."

I grabbed a notepad from my purse, crossing out "hamburger" and "apples" and hurriedly scribbling "glucose," "glycogen," "GSD type III," and "healthy liver versus ???" I would call Carol Morrison in the morning.

"Dr. Marris, what can Martin and I *do*?" I was not going to cry. I had to stay calm, think, get information. I felt as though I were pulling details painstakingly from Dr. Marris. Didn't he realize he was my lifeline to hope? To information? To . . . everything?

"I will schedule Sammy's needle biopsy to be performed in the next week or so. In the meantime, get some Argo cornstarch. I want you to stir two teaspoons into each baby food feeding and do the same with Sammy's formula each time, shaking well. Don't cook the cornstarch and mix it up fresh. Do this with every single feeding. I want you to feed Sammy *every three hours*."

Argo cornstarch? For a condition that was as rare as GSD? Good grief. I had cornstarch in my pantry, along with Pillsbury Best flour.

Dr. Marris continued. "I want to see you and Sammy one week after the needle biopsy is performed. We'll go through the biopsy and see how Sammy is doing on the cornstarch therapy."

The doctor stood up, signaling that we were done. I scribbled "Argo cornstarch—why?" on my pad, collected Sammy, and thanked Dr. Marris for helping us figure out what was wrong with my baby.

"Oh. One last thing. Where can I go for more information or help?" I had no idea where to turn.

"You can contact NORD, the National Organization for Rare Disorders. The front desk can give you the number." And off went Dr. Marris, striding into the grayness of the hospital hallway.

Well, so much for a local support group or hands-on information. However, it was a start in figuring out Sammy's condition.

Sammy and I wandered back through the perky waiting room of the genetics department. Our little friend by the spinny wheel had disappeared. New tired-eyed parents and sickly kids filled the waiting room. I remember looking at them, realizing that we were *one of them*, now. A family with GSD. Not too different from a family with diabetes, with lupus, with cystic fibrosis, with Down syndrome. Several million of us hunting for help, for information.

We hit Pak 'N Save on the way home, buying boxes of Argo cornstarch and several jars of Gerber bean-and-bacon toddler food. I felt like Captain Jean-Luc Picard on *Star Trek*'s *Enterprise*, bolstered with fierce determination as I thought, *Engage*. The only problem was, I really didn't know where I was going. I had no map, just a tiny bit of information wrestled from the doctor.

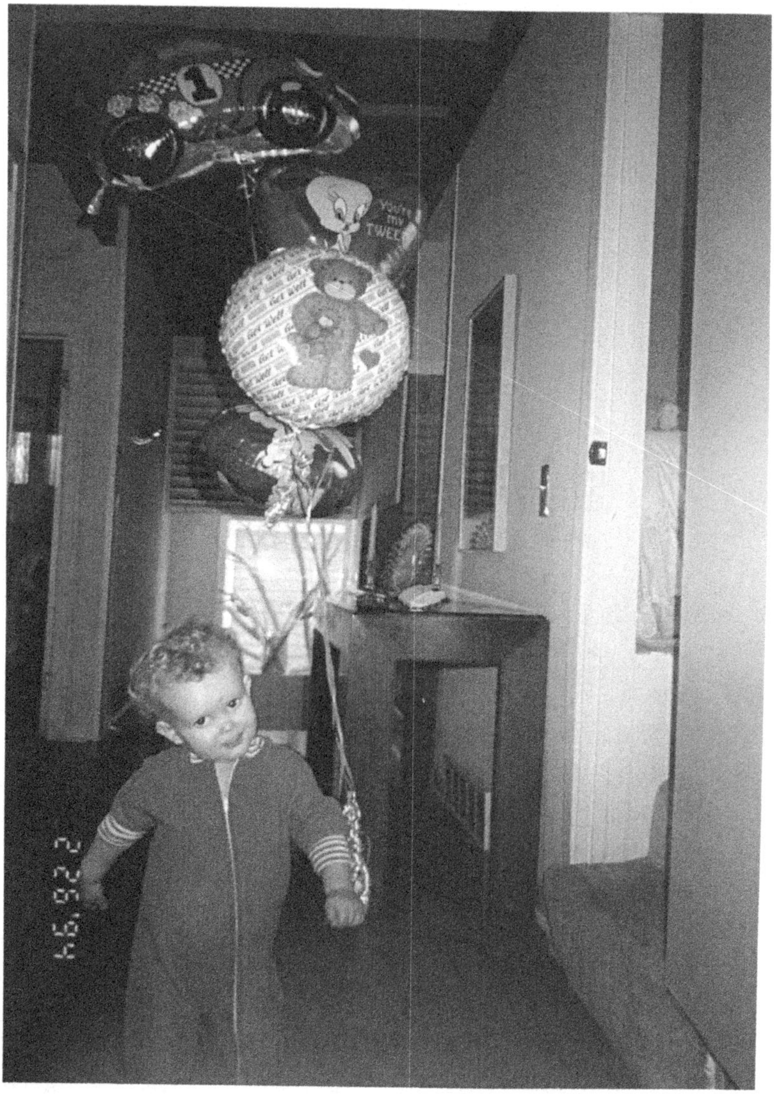

The big two

10

So, What's "Normal"?

That night, I created a cornstarch drawer, cleared a cornstarch shelf, and taped a cornstarch dosing schedule on the fridge.

I found a huge Tupperware bowl and dumped two boxes of Argo cornstarch in it. That night, because it was Tuesday, we most likely had meat loaf, mashed potatoes, and broccoli. I sneakily stirred one teaspoon of cornstarch into Sammy's potatoes to test the waters.

At the dinner table, we hashed over the day's events. Martin had gotten budget approval to build out more lab space at his work, because Cardizem, a new heart drug, was selling like hotcakes. Tee was excited because he got to handle worms in his science class, and "they were gooshy and they pooped on you." I felt a bit hopeful for the first time in months. I briefed the guys on the findings with Dr. Marris, trying to remember the connection between the liver, glycogen, and glucose. I glanced at Sammy sideways to see if he'd eat the potatoes.

No problem. The potatoes went down and the meat loaf did too.

"So, we've got to feed Sammy every three hours and mix raw cornstarch into his food and formula. No, I don't understand why exactly, except that Dr. Marris said it would help keep Sam's blood sugar up between feedings. Blood sugar is also called glucose, Dr. Marris said. Sammy hasn't been walking because with low blood sugar, he's just so tired." I patted Sammy's arm, gooey with meat loaf gravy. "Now, Sammy, the doctor told us today that your liver doesn't work quite like Mom's or Dad's or Tee's."

"I know. It's right here," replied Sammy, patting his tummy where his liver lay. "It's kinda big." He had been paying attention to every word Dr. Marris had said earlier that day.

"Well, if you start to feel tired, you tell Dad or Mom or Tee right away, okay? Dr. Marris says that cornstarch will keep you from feeling so worn out, and it will help you grow strong. We'll help you take it every three hours. I know it doesn't taste like mac and cheese, but it's not too bad." I went to the kitchen and brought out a little bowlful to show Sammy. He stuck two fingers in it and dabbed, making a fluff of snow on the table. I stuck my fingers in the bowl, too, licking off some of the powder. "See? This is what we use to make Oobleck, the fun white clay stuff. It's pretty cool that *this* will make you feel better."

"Okay," replied Sammy, very matter-of-factly about this new culinary turn of events. "I liked the play wall at Dr. Marris's with the spinny wheel. I met a new friend there, but she couldn't talk."

This was day one of Sammy's treatment plan. Supplies, organization, and family communication. Within days, Sammy learned to come to us and say, "I'm cornstarch tired."

***

Looking back at that night at the dinner table, I think about how I introduced Sammy's chronic illness to him. "Your liver doesn't work quite like Mom's or Dad's. Cornstarch will help you to grow and not feel tired." Did I tell Sammy too much or too little that night? I had taken twenty-four hours of psych classes in college, but I felt unprepared to deal with the GSD diagnosis. Dr. Marris just didn't "get" how lost I felt as a parent. He was a scientist, not a therapist. Our family had no one to tell us what to do—certainly not the geneticist with his steely eyes. It was 1993, and the first internet search engine had emerged, but most of us relied on phone calls, books, faxes, and personal contacts for information. That's all we had to go on with Sam's rare condition. That, and a telephone number for NORD.

In the early twentieth century, parents thought that their offspring had no cognition abilities until they started to speak; they were just miniature, empty-headed adults. Then, psychologist Jean Piaget hypothesized that nothing could be farther from the truth. Childhood cognitive development follows four general stages, according to Piaget. At birth through about age two, a child explores his world through the five senses and by touching objects or by putting them into the mouth. By age two through seven, the child will develop imagination and memory. He will conceive of the present and the past and begin to understand symbols. *Tomorrow,* he understands, he will go to McDonald's, pictured in his mind as the "Golden Arches" or the Ronald McDonald statue. The symbols represent a Happy Meal, a toy surprise, and a playscape to the child. And "tomorrow" means "not now." As the child becomes seven to about eleven, he understands that he is not the center of the universe. In other words, his playmate Timmy may want the blue Tonka truck and not want to share it. By age eleven and beyond, the child can use logic to solve problems and plan for the future.[1] Hmmmm. Dad says no, so go to Mom, right?

When I first told Sammy about his condition, he was nearly two years old; in other words, he was capable of understanding just a bit about his liver with a physical *touch* to his tummy and *imagining* that the "thing" inside the tummy somehow made him strong or weak. Considering Sammy's probable development stage, it was most likely useful for him to also *touch and taste* the cornstarch that he would consume every three hours to control his blood-sugar level, because that learning technique was using the child's senses.

Two-year-old Sammy could also begin to make an association between a lack of cornstarch and tiredness. However, he couldn't conceptualize *how* the cornstarch worked, or *how* the liver processed foods. For that matter, neither could I. Additionally, Sammy couldn't conceptualize the idea of "illness," especially not "chronic illness." Most likely, the child's first perceptions of his GSD evolved from Dr. Marris's actions and our first matter-of-fact family dinner conversation. Our tears, our uncertainties—they crawled out after our two kids were safely in bed. Somehow, Martin and I knew that we had to be calm and factual in front of our boys.

---

1. "4 Cognitive Stages for Child Development," Learning RX, accessed January 28, 2020, https://www.learningrx.com/4-cognitive-stages-for-child-development.

11

Surgery Ahead

"Help, Carol!" I had called my pediatrician friend after I put Sam down for a nap. I had taken another personal day to regroup my thoughts about a week after we had met with Dr. Marris. I was a snarled mess of emotions.

We had gone cornstarch wild in our house after the visit with the geneticist, stirring in two teaspoons for a 3:00 a.m. feeding, as well as 6:00 a.m., 9:00 a.m., and so on. It was literally every three hours. Sammy seemed nonplussed over the new routine. "How do you feel today?" I asked him several times the first three days of the new schedule.

"Okay, Mama. Can we go to Jumpin' Johnnie's Play Pit? And will you get me a new book at Borders for Valemtime's Day? [Sammy's word for the holiday as he understood it] They have cappuccino there. I like cappuccino."

Sam wasn't kiddin'. He *did* like cappuccino. (And this word he pronounced perfectly!) Martin and I had often taken the kids to Borders on a sleety winter's day to buy a couple of books. Sam would end up with us at the coffee bar, one chubby leg crossed over the other, sipping his cappuccino in a debonair manner. Age two going on forty.

"Well, Tee will be home from school in three hours. Retha will get him so you and I can play after your nap. We'll go to Jumpin' Johnnie's on Saturday with Tee, because you're being such a good boy today!"

As Sammy's breathing became regular during his nap, I dialed Carol quickly. "Carol. This is Janet and guess what! We got in to see Dr. Marris. He thinks Sam has a recessive genetic condition called glycogen storage disease. He doesn't know which kind yet, but I got a call earlier about the needle biopsy at Children's Mercy. Yes, it's a week from Tuesday. You know, I've never heard of this GSD. Have you? Oh—you have? In medical school? A page somewhere in one of your textbooks? Well, Dr. Marris used a bunch of words I didn't know at the time—like 'glucose' and 'glycogen.' My Webster's dictionary doesn't really tell me much. For Pete's sake, I don't even know about healthy blood sugar. I just remember that with both pregnancies, I had to watch my sugar intake. With Sammy, I absolutely craved fruit juices my entire pregnancy."

Carol replied in her most soothing, doctorly voice. "My kids are still at school, so I'll scoot over and bring you some of my medical school textbooks that I have at home. I'll mark some passages on GSD and on blood-sugar control. You can start learning about Sammy's condition."

Maybe knowledge would be power, as they say. Maybe knowledge would calm the feeling in my gut. Maybe I would feel just a bit in control of the situation.

Biopsy day came. I had been diligent with Sammy's cornstarch routine, and it seemed to be helping—helping a lot. It was as if the child's little inner computer were booting up and coming alive. Sammy was alert and happy, cruising down the family room couch with Barney the dinosaur in hand, much like we had attempted months ago with physical therapy. It was a darn cornstarch miracle. Argo was my new savior.

On surgery day, Martin, Sammy, and I headed to Children's Mercy Hospital, while Retha drove Tee to school. Our freckled boy wonder clutched a "body box" school project that Martin had helped him with the night before. The box was anatomically correct, with objects from Hobby Lobby wired and glued into the recesses to *sort of* look like the liver, kidneys, rib cage, spleen, and heart. I had raced through Hobby Lobby two days prior like Peyton Manning, tossing into my cart stuffed fabric fruits and any other object that might look like a body part. We knew Tee's friend Jimmy was going to have the best body box in the class, and sure enough, he did. There were flowing veins of "blood" circulating all through his body box, and a pulsing "heart." Not fair. Jimmy's dad was a cardiologist. Lunch that day was going to be "a body-part buffet"—carrot sticks for fingers, Jell-O for intestines, and peeled grapes for eyeballs. "It's going to be gross!" Tee told Martin enthusiastically. When you are seven, gross and gooshy are wonderful things.

The scheduling nurse at Children's Mercy had told us "no food" before the procedure, because Sam would undergo a general anesthesia. I noticed that on the way to the hospital, Sam's head lolled to one side of the car seat. We carried him into the surgery waiting room, a floppy doll. Were we supposed to have skipped food and cornstarch? Well, the surgery nurse had said so, and we were rule followers.

After about an hour and a half, we headed back to recovery. Sam was wailing loudly, hooked up to a heart monitor, an IV bag dripping glucose into him. The beeping equipment was terrifying; Sammy was beet red, writhing in the hospital bed, a nurse stroking his arm. "The type of anesthesia used in this procedure usually makes kids very anxious and angry," the recovery room nurse informed me. Yes, Sammy was angry—absolutely screaming out of control. I leaned over and kissed his sweaty forehead. I felt so guilty—we had just put our son through a tough procedure. The child had already been scanned, poked, and stuck multiple times in his young life. He had been to five different specialists thus far, averaging about three appointments a week since the liver ultrasound a few months ago. However, Dr. Marris had said we needed to know what type of GSD Sammy had. The symptoms and treatment were different for each type, and we had to manage the condition properly.

The surgeon came into the room in the midst of the screaming chaos.

"We've completed a percutaneous liver biopsy on Sammy. I inserted a thin tube through his abdomen and took a small tissue sample.[1] Pathology will analyze this sample to determine what type of GSD Sammy has. We should have some information for you both in about three to five days." Duty done, the surgeon smiled encouragingly at us and headed out the door, tapping the doorframe with his palm authoritatively, as if to say, *That's that.*

That *wasn't* that. The tissue sample taken was too small. It came back as "inconclusive for GSD type." Two months later, at Dr. Marris's strong encouragement, Sammy went through another needle biopsy, screaming just as vigorously. This time, we found out that Sammy had GSD 1a, often called Von Gierke disease. It was more serious.

***

"GSD 1a is technically a glucose-phosphatase deficiency. In

---

1. "Liver Biopsy," Mayo Clinic, November 24, 2020, https://www.mayoclinic.org/tests-procedures/liverbiopsy/about/pac-20394576.

individuals with this condition, the glucose-6-enzyme is either missing or malfunctioning."[2]

It was 10:30 on a Monday night. Martin and I had supervised showers and stories. The dishwasher whirred and the coffeepot blinked at us, saying, *"I'll have the black magic ready for you tomorrow at 5:15 a.m."* I had thrown in a load of laundry and settled at my desk, poring over one of Carol Morrison's medical textbooks. I found there the same sort of information that today is a Google away, how GSD is "a malfunction of the catalytic subunit (G6Pse) which characterizes GSD 1a. . . . G6Pse is a nine-helical endoplasmic reticulum transmembrane protein. . . ."[3]

I sighed, flipping to the next page of Carol's book and rubbing my tired eyes. None of it made any sense to me. The only words I understood in the text were "a," "the," and "malfunction." *Malfunction.* Such a tidy, scientific word for the real mess our family was in. Malfunction? Sammy's entire body didn't work right. *Malfunction*? Would Sammy ever *walk*? My mind couldn't go to those dark, what-if thoughts.

I turned to textbook two, discouraged and fighting rising panic. More of the same kind of inscrutable sentences, like: "Glycogen storage disease type I (GSDI) is characterized by accumulation of excessive glycogen and fat in the liver and kidneys that can result in an enlarged liver and kidneys and growth retardation leading to short stature."[4] All I saw was "enlarged liver and kidneys . . . growth retardation . . . short stature." Oh, my God. Would Sammy always be child sized? What would happen with an enlarged liver? I started to visualize cherub-cheeked Sammy, only four feet tall with a pouch

---

2. Jeng-Jer Shieh et al., "The Molecular Basis of Glycogen Storage Disease Type 1a," *Journal of Biological Chemistry* 277, no. 7 (February 2002): 5047, https://doi.org/10.1074/jbc.M110486200.
3. Kathleen R. Ruddiman and Catherine Anastasopoulou, "Type 1a Glycogen Storage Disease Treatment & Management," Medscape, July 7, 2021, emedicine.medscape.com/article/119318-treatment#d8.
4. Ruddiman and Anastasopoulou, "Type 1a Glycogen Storage Disease."

collecting urine. Would this be his future? My panic took off big-time.

Focus, Janet. Focus. You can read this. You have *to read this.* I heaved open my huge Merriam-Webster dictionary. All right. "Stored glycogen." Mr. Webster told me that meant stored carbohydrates in body tissues. Well, *that* I could understand, but what would that *do* to the body? "Glucose," I read from Carol's book, determined to understand Sammy's condition. Again, Mr. Webster informed: "An important energy source . . . part of many carbohydrates." I looked at my scribbled list from a few days prior: "autosomal recessive genetic disorder." I remembered that Dr. Marris told me that Martin and I each carried the recessive gene that caused mutations in Sammy. I flipped through the dictionary faster, as though my urgency could somehow fix Sammy's predicament. "Autosomal recessive"—that was a medical term that meant when Sammy was conceived, he had to get two copies of the abnormal gene for his GSD to manifest. He did, one from each parent. Sammy had GSD in every cell of his body. Tee, the older brother, had beaten the 25 percent roll of the dice.

My eyes traveled back to the ominous medical-book entry. "Enlarged liver, growth retardation, and short stature." The hope that had wavered after my visit with Dr. Marris evaporated. *Will Sammy always have an enlarged liver? Will he spend his life as short, as different? Will he ever meet a girl? How could he go on a date, lugging his cornstarch? My kid has to have a "normal" life,* I thought, angry at what fate had thrown at us. *This is not how life is supposed to work. I've gotta fix this. I've gotta fix this.*

Discouraged, with a churning gut, I turned out the desk light, checked on Tee and Sammy, and rolled into bed. The 3:00 a.m. alarm for Sammy's cornstarch would come very soon.

PART 2

BABY STEPS

12

Control Freak

As the weeks passed, our family settled into a "somewhat normal" routine: after all, we were now a *GSD* family. We all, in a sense, had to manage this chronic condition. Martin and I kept on the rigorous cornstarch schedule, determined to give Sammy every chance. Sam responded like a textbook case, I think, had we been able to *find* a textbook case. I had read in one of Carol's medical books that before cornstarch was discovered as a way to maintain blood sugar, kids died from GSD. Apparently, the cornstarch discovery had only been since the mid-1970s. There were very few living adult humans with GSD to actually study. It was a new and scary frontier. And we were on that frontier, kicking and screaming, lost, scared.

At some point in Sammy's early diagnosis, I read a beautiful memoir that pinged my heart. The memoir, *Raising Henry*, examines a mother's role in raising a child with Down syndrome, otherwise known as trisomy 21. Unlike glycogen storage disease, Down syndrome is fairly common, impacting about one out of seven hundred births across all races. The extra twenty-first chromosome consists of over three hundred genes, creating a massive genetic puzzle. Children with Down syndrome must cope with reduced mental capacity, low muscle tone, sensory imbalances, eating and swallowing difficulties, and heart defects.

My takeaway from *Raising Henry* was that parenting a child with special needs is a continuous battle of investigation, of learning. Fortunately, with some chronic illnesses and disabilities such as Down syndrome and type 1 diabetes, support systems in the US are numerous. I must admit I was a bit jealous when I read that when Henry left the hospital as a newborn, the mother, Rachel, was put in contact with an agency that would coordinate intervention services. The well-educated family would receive a team of therapists to help Henry work on physical and cognitive development. At present, early intervention for Down syndrome is mandated by federal law, but the resources are distributed on the state level. As Henry's mother writes, Down syndrome children from Colorado may be put on a waiting list; families from New Jersey pay for services on a sliding scale. The mom and little Henry were lucky to live in New York state. In her family's case, the state charged the family's insurance and subsequently made up any costs not covered by insurance. In New York, uninsured children are totally covered by the early intervention program. In poorer states with less tax revenue, the intervention programs are not as robust, entailing waiting lists. Meanwhile, the Down syndrome child and family manage as best they can, operating in the dark. Man, I could relate to that situation. Whether it's Down syndrome or cystic fibrosis or GSD, we're all pretty much in the same boat.

When our family finally got Sammy diagnosed at twenty-one months, our "intervention program" was a slip of paper with the phone number for NORD. That was it. Martin and I knew little about how to nurture Sammy or what to expect of him developmentally. Part of the issue with Sammy was that Mother Nature dealt him a rare disorder, affecting about one in one hundred thousand births. Research didn't exist for early intervention when Sammy was born in 1992, because children with GSD had only just begun to survive. Most physicians could vaguely remember studying GSD in medical school.

Dr. Marris at Children's Mercy Hospital finally gave us the name of a child nearby in Shawnee, Kansas, who had GSD 1a. I think I had badgered the man into submission by our third appointment. Sammy was about twenty-four months by this time, and I called to arrange a meeting with the family. One Sunday afternoon, the Hayles family eagerly met the Sawyers.

Twelve-year-old Billy Sawyer came racing into his home, wiping his sweaty face on his red-striped tee shirt. He had been out playing soccer. I was so relieved: here was a boy with GSD who was simply out playing with his friends. Perhaps Sammy could ride a bike, swim, go to high school, go on a date someday. Right now, all Martin and I were seeing was Sammy vigorously crawling across our family room floor. Possibilities opened up to me like two prayerful hands cupped upward. As Billy gulped down a glass of water, his mom, Grace, filled two large syringes with cornstarch and water, fitting a nasogastric tube on the end of one of the syringes. I'm sure I stood flabbergasted as Billy maneuvered the NG tube up his nose, down through his esophagus, and into his stomach, compressing the attached syringe and releasing the starch into his stomach. He grabbed the second syringe, fitted it onto the NG tubing, and squeezed again. Billy handed the syringes and NG tube back to Grace with a "Bye, Mom," and zoomed out the door to his buddies. The cornstarch routine was just that—routine to Billy.

Hope lifted us up that afternoon as we drove home.

***

One day while we were still fairly new at GSD care, I headed down the stairs after work to the family room. It had been a doozie of a day. One department member came to me upset, thinking she should get to go to more training seminars each year. At her job level, company policy allowed her two per year; she insisted on four, harrumphing out of my office with a glare that nearly seared my eyebrows. The 1099-INTs didn't print off in the computer room, either. A programming problem. We had to get it figured out, because federal law mandated that the INTs had to be mailed on January 31, and today was January 28. Fifty thousand employees were waiting on us, and we had two days. Two days. Massive fines would smack the company if our department couldn't get the tax forms figured out. On top of all this, I had heard rumblings of a new merger with our company. Oh, good grief. That merger meant that my department would have to either assimilate or add benefit plans. That merger, so glamorous on paper, would entail endless meetings with our legal department, Ernst and Young consulting, and company programmers. Voluminous communications. Hand-holding the shareholders. Benefit-plan tweaking. The drama never ended, but it was also oddly exhilarating. Come feast and famine, war and peace, snow and blazing heat—you didn't mess with employees' benefits.

As I stepped into the family room, I met Retha, who was breathless. It was only the second time I'd ever seen her *breathless.*

"Just ten minutes ago, Sammy took four steps! He was cruising down the couch and saw Barney over by the coffee table and went for him. Four steps!"

I was thrilled but so envious. Retha had witnessed something Martin and I had been waiting on for the last five months. And I had missed it. What was I doing, going to work every day? How could benefit plans ever compare to Sammy's first steps? Did I have to choose my work over my child? Why couldn't I have both?

That night: joy. Sammy took more steps for Martin and me. Tee, my freckled bundle of energy, had said to Sammy, "If you walk over to me, I'll give you a booster-jet ride in your dee dee." And so, Sam simply walked to big brother and gave him a hug.

***

The next day, I stood in the copy room, my feet aching from my navy heels. I absently ran off copies of executive deferred-compensation plans, looking up at the bulletin board in angst. The 1099 form problem had been solved, but I was bone tired, or as my grandma Julia used to say, I was all out of spizerinck-tom. I'd gotten up with Sammy for his 3:00 a.m. feeding, then back up again at 5:15 a.m. to shower and dress for work. The "every three hours" grind of GSD had gotten to me. Martin was flying back and forth to Paris for his latest project, and so Retha and I had to power through the weeks. Would I ever understand Sammy's condition? Would I ever feel like I could get my arms around all the chaos at work? And then—I looked up, and there it was on the bulletin board. It was a message, I think, for me.

Footprints in the Sand

One night I dreamed I was walking
along the beach with the Lord.
Many scenes from my life flashed across
the sky.
In each scene I noticed footprints in the
sand.

Sometimes there were two sets of
  footprints,
other times there were one set of
  footprints.

. . .

"The times when you have
seen only one set of footprints,
is when I carried you."

—Mary Stevenson[1]

"It was then that I carried you." The words felt like a warm, comforting hand on my shoulder, and unprofessional tears fell onto my stack of copies. I remember my sense of desperation contrasted with an extreme moment of peace. I knew that God wouldn't sweep in and "fix" Sammy. There were no guarantees that Sammy would get better. There were no guarantees that my work would settle down. Life was, well, life. Life was Georgie chasing after Tee as he somersaulted across the backyard. Life was feeding the goats at Children's Farmstead in Overland Park with the boys. Life was that stolen moment of wine with Martin after a day shredded of any semblance of order. Life was spit-up on my shoes and baby crap on my sleeve.

Well, control freak, I thought that day, *let go. You don't* have *life; it* has *you.*

***

Sammy seemed to be taking his new medical condition with childlike calmness. Two weeks after his first steps, he trotted

1. Mary Stevenson, "Footprints in the Sand," Footprints in the Sand, accessed August 11, 2022, https://footprintssandpoem.com/mary-stevenson-version-of-footprints-in-the-sand/.

Barney the dinosaur for short walks all over the house: on the couch, the coffee table, the stairs. "Barney, we'll go to the park with the twisty-turny slide tomorrow. But, Barney, you have to put your toys away first. Here. In this red bucket. Don't let me tell you twice. And it will be time for your cornstarch soon." The words just exploded out of that child.

I, however, wasn't taking Sammy's medical condition as well as he.

Control and discipline have always governed my life. They create my white picket fence that keeps everything mentally corralled. Even when I was four, I had my Little Golden Book collection sorted neatly. My Barbie dolls sat in a row on my bedroom shelf, followed by my green-haired troll dolls, tallest to shortest. As an adult, my clothes closet was arranged by color, with subcategories of summer versus winter, and sub-subcategories of short-sleeved versus long-sleeved. My spice rack was alphabetized from allspice to wasabi. I had my MBA, and I flossed nightly. Check. Check. Check.

In my twenties, I felt like I had life by the tail. I was taught in childhood that with education and hard work, you could get what you wanted in life. If that didn't work, you'd grab onto your situation like a pit bull with a dead squirrel, shake it, and work some more until you got what you wanted. You stayed *on plan*. If you didn't succeed at life, you were lazy or inefficient.

I came by control and discipline naturally. Mom and Dad were both teachers. They had met in 1950 at Hutchinson High School in Kansas. Dad was teaching typing and shorthand there, while Mom taught English and ran the school newspaper. Story goes, Dad met Mom at a faculty school picnic, as Mom, dark haired and skinny, was in the food line heaping raw carrots and celery onto her paper plate. Dad wowed her with a real pickup line: "You don't like carrots much, do you?" The magic flowed, and Mom and Dad got married in 1952. I arrived, quite conveniently, 363 days later. Right on plan, of course.

I don't remember much of Hutchinson but more of Emporia, Kansas. We had moved there when I was six, because Dad had gotten a finance teaching position at the state university. Mom easily got an English teaching position at a small Presbyterian college just a mile from our home.

Life was tranquil and predictable in Emporia. On Sunday mornings, Mom would pop a roast into her blue speckled pan before church, dumping in peeled potatoes and carrots and two cans of beer for tenderness. Weekdays were a rush, with a glass of Tang for breakfast and Rice Krispies cereal with whole milk. Monday was meat loaf, green beans, and baked potato night. But, on Thursdays, Mom would buy Swanson chicken pot pies at Kroger—four for a dollar. They'd bubble for an hour in the oven, the crust turning a magical tan. When I'd cut into a pot pie, I'd hear the little "pffft" of hot air escape, the creamy gravy spilling onto my plate.

You see, Thursday night was choir practice at the Congregational church down the road. Mom reckoned that the pot pie shortcut was okay since we had to rush out of the house at 6:45 p.m. I'd sit in the front pew at the church as the choir hashed and rehashed "Seek Ye the Lord." Dad had a solo part: anxiety sweat would run down his face as I would read Nancy Drew mysteries like *The Secret of the Old Clock*.

When I was growing up, Dad *always* retreated to his office in the basement after supper to prepare for his 7:30 a.m. managerial finance class. Mom *always* had a clipboard full of themes to grade, her red stick pen placed neatly across the top page. Every Saturday, Dad would cut the grass or tackle small repair work. Mom would get her hair "done" into an impregnable helmet of dark brown curls and then head to Kroger. I would clean our two-bedroom ranch to a spit shine with Pledge furniture polish, singing at the top of my lungs to

"Eight Days a Week." The Beatles. To a twelve-year-old, they were good-lookin' and glamorous.

Several times a year, Mom would decide to treat Dad to a homemade pie. The raisin pie efforts had fizzled after Mom's two-year desperate bake-a-thon. Dad would be out on a stepladder in the Kansas fall glory, wearing paint-splattered khakis. He'd hang his old transistor radio on the top rung of the ladder, painting the house sideboard vigorously and listening to Kansas University football, his alma mater. His favorite game was KU against Oklahoma, the big rival. "Dammit! Come on, KU," Dad would holler at the radio, slapping the paintbrush against the siding of the house. "Dammit, KU! *Run!*"

Mom would come into the backyard during the stream of curses and say, "Steve, I think I'll make a pie. What kind would you like?"

"Uh, I think I'd like cherry." Dad *always* asked for cherry. Every time.

I don't think my parents meant to be so precise, so disciplined. They couldn't escape their childhoods, any more than I can escape mine to this day.

My dad was born in 1922, the union of a Congregationalist minister, John Butcher, and the organist at a church in Leavenworth, Kansas, Lillian Heath. Grandpa John had lost his first wife, and when he was age fifty, the lovely Miss Lillian caught his eye as she filled the church with "Faith of Our Fathers." Lillian made the pipe organ at the church absolutely rumble, and most certainly did the same to Reverend Butcher's heart. The woman was both pretty and smart. She had graduated from Beloit College in Wisconsin in 1918 and had gone on to the Kansas City Conservatory of Music, where she majored in the pipe organ. At age thirty-two, Lillian was considered a spinster, but the reverend changed all that. The two married in 1921, calming the wagging tongues in Leavenworth, and moved to Hutchinson, Kansas, to a larger church. In 1922, my dad—the blond, curly-headed Stevie—was born. He was a gift, for Lillian had been thirty-three when she became pregnant in 1921.

Life does twist. We know this intellectually. When it happens, however, it stabs our gut because it's not really supposed to happen to *us*. And, true to life's twists, in 1929 as the Great Depression was erupting, Reverend Butcher caught pneumonia and died. Lillian was left with the parsonage, a tiny pension, and seven-year-old Stevie.

Years later, as I read Grandma's diary about my dad, I could see why *my* mom always took care of him—just like Lillian had taken care of Dad as a child. I could see why my dad was an uncertain, anxious adult. His father and comfortable life were ripped from him in the middle of the Great Depression. Lillian raised Stevie while baking cinnamon rolls to sell out of her home. She played the organ at McPherson's Mortuary in Hutchinson. They got by. They barely got by.

With one foot planted figuratively on my dad's backside, Lillian hustled him into a local community college after high school. After serving in World War II, Dad worked summers at Sears, Roebuck and Company, selling lawn equipment and paying his way through a BS in finance at the University of Kansas. Later, when he was teaching at Hutchinson High School, Dad would take summer school business classes for his master's degree at Pittsburg State. Lillian's foot on the backside then switched over to my mom's foot. In 1960, as Dad moved to an assistant professorship at Emporia State University, he began postgraduate coursework in finance at Indiana University in Bloomington, Indiana. Doggedly, Dad would teach Introduction to Corporate Finance and Management during the school year in Emporia. Mom would teach Shakespeare, steadily plowing her way through a stack of student themes each week. Every summer, for six years, my family would drive five hundred miles to Bloomington, where we sweltered in married-student housing. I'd play kickball and jacks with all the other kids whose daddies were in school. After dinner, I'd work through my weekly pile of library books. We had no television, no telephone—just a main room, a bathroom, and a tiny kitchen. I'd fall asleep at night on a cot in our apartment, just inches away from Dad's desk. I'd hear the soft flip-flip of pages as Dad pored over macroeconomics. The window-box fan whirred and sucked in the wet-blanket-ness of Bloomington air. Mom typed up Dad's papers on the thirty-pound Smith Corona typewriter. Peck-peck-peck-zing! She was fast.

When I think about my mom, she was no slouch, either. Mom's father, George Malcolm, was an attorney in Pittsburg, Kansas. Julia was a legal secretary at his law firm, and at age thirty-two, she made George's torts tingle. Marriage came soon after. My mom, Jeanne, was born the next year in 1920, followed in five years by sister Janet.

The Great Depression years were not as tough on the Malcolm family as on most. Even in the midst of a crisis, the townspeople of Pittsburg still needed an attorney. Grandpa George would settle a drunk-driving charge in court, and soon, two cases of fine local wine from Chanute would arrive on the front porch of his home. When Grandpa George helped Lonnie Garner with his furniture store's mortgage issues, Lonnie gave the family a beautiful forest-green area rug for the living room.

Mom went to Pittsburg State College as an undergrad. I still don't know how, but she ended up at Northwestern, obtaining a master's in English with a 4.0. By age twenty-two, she was teaching English in Ellsworth, Kansas, moving a few years later to the big town of Hutchinson. "Ellsworth is at the damn ends of the world," Mom would often say to Dad. In Ellsworth, you could go to a bar, go fishing, or go to church.

Mom broke rules. When she and Dad got married in

Hutchinson, she kept teaching at the high school, and local tongues flapped. *Did your husband lose his job? Are you in money trouble?* Blue-haired ladies would pepper Mom with questions in the checkout line of Dillon's grocery. When Mom got pregnant with me precisely as planned, Hutchinson really talked. The high school suspended Mom's teaching contract because she was beginning to "show." "The kids can't see a pregnant lady teaching them verbs," the principal explained to Mom, as though her growing midsection would lead the high school kids to rampant sex in the halls. When I was a year old, Mom went back to teaching—this time geometry, as the school math teacher had inopportunely died in the middle of the school year. I stayed with Mrs. Prop next door, a widow woman (another Kansas expression!) who radiated love and smelled like chocolate chip cookies. Again, the town yapped: *Jeanne, you're taking a man's job. Why are you doing this? Why aren't you home with your child? Are you both in financial trouble?* Mom just had to work; she was so damn smart. Dirty diapers were no match for congruent triangles. I get that.

Virginia Nicholson in *Perfect Wives in Ideal Homes* writes about the era I grew up in. The 1940s represented a time of war and privation, while the 1960s began to blow apart traditions. The 1950s? Well, they were a forgotten decade until recently. Only 1.2 percent of women actually went to a university at this time, Nicholson estimates.[2] In the midst of the fifties, my mom just didn't fit: she was educated and career oriented.

I am a true product of my past. As the poem "Footprints" settled into my heart that day in the copy room at work, I realized that instead of the control and discipline I had learned as a kid, life was full of uncertain turns and a series of choices, especially with a chronically ill child. Should I work

---

2. Juliet Gardiner, "The Story of Women in the 1950s," *History Today* 65, no. 9 (September 9, 2015), https://www.historytoday.com/reviews/story-women-1950s.

outside the home, or stay home with the children? Could I do a little of each? I remember grabbing up my stack of deferred-compensation data that day and heading to my desk to scribble out a quick pro-con list for myself. Fifteen minutes later, I rolled my chair back from my desk. There it was: a chicken scratch of alternatives.

The pros of continuing work were several. First off, I listed financial security and insurance. That was so important with a child—especially an ill one. Then, there was the exhilaration of using my brain: solving those accounting problems or delivering an impactful benefits presentation. And then, the Big One: my ego. I wanted and I *needed* to feel intelligent and live out my dream as a career woman. I had grown up surrounded by an aura of education and careers. It's just *what you did as a woman. Anything less was subpar.*

My pro list for becoming a stay-at-home mom was equally strong. Unfortunately, internet systems in 1998 didn't provide work-at-home capabilities. Amazon Prime and Whole Foods didn't exist to deliver the endless demand of diapers, cereal, and hamburger to my home. Plus, my boss was a traditionalist. My department needed *one* manager in the office—not job sharing. And that manager had to be there physically, five to six days a week.

So. Working from home in 1998 or job sharing was just not an option for me. I dealt with an either-or situation. What would staying at home mean for me?

My heart told me that staying at home meant I could see those precious boys more. As a working mom, I heard a lot of buzz about "quality time with my children." *Shouldn't all my time be quality time?* I wondered. Also, if I stayed at home, I could pull the stress load off Martin. We could have great home-cooked meals, or at least home-cooked meals. Martin and I could have time to talk at the end of the day, instead of falling into an exhausted stupor at ten thirty each night.

I could be at all the boys' activities. I could take the time to train, really train Sammy to understand and manage his condition. I thought back to all the mother-daughter tea events at my middle school, so many years ago. My mom could never come because of her teaching schedule. Each year, I felt like an abandoned orphan at the tea. It just hurt. Did I ever want my boys to feel that sense of loss?

13

Dear Mom

Mom and I wrote to each other once a week. We only lived one hundred miles apart, but long-distance calls were for emergencies only. You called when someone had died, was dying, or was going to die. One time when Mom actually called me, her poodle Nicki had gone to the great kennel in the sky. Another time, I picked up the phone, a bit anxious when I saw Mom's area code.

"Hey, Mom. What's up?"

"Could I stay with you and Martin for a week or two?" Mom never bothered with chitchat. Her voice was measured and even.

"Of course! We'd love it. Is Dad coming too?" Mom and Dad were always together, like Mutt and Jeff.

"Well, he's coming from Emporia to the University of Kansas Medical Center by ambulance. He had a heart attack and is in Newman Hospital in Emporia. He's being transferred to KU Med, and the doctors think he will need a quadruple bypass. Your house is only forty minutes from KU Med, and I may need to camp out for a while."

"Oh, good grief! When did this happen?" I felt like I had been slapped. This couldn't be real.

"Yesterday morning. Steve was eating breakfast and then started having chest pain. I called an ambulance and got him over to Newman Hospital in Emporia. Thank God it's only a mile away. He's being transferred to KU tomorrow."

It had been hours and hours, and Mom had finally called. Dad had had a major heart attack, and I had to pry the information out of her. *Oh, good grief, Mom. How could you be so calm in this situation?*

***

> Dear Mom,
>
> I'm so glad Dad is back home and that his heart is doing well. I know you loved being with the grandkids for the past three weeks, but being at the hospital all day was tough on you, I bet. Sammy and Tee say, "Hugs to Grandma B!"
>
> Sammy and I had another appointment with Dr. Marris yesterday. I bombarded him with a new set of questions about GSD. At the end of our appointment, he looked at me over his glasses and had the nerve to say to me, "You ask a lot of questions, don't you?"
>
> Well, Mom, I didn't want to anger our only GSD expert. I just gave Dr. Marris my best withering teacher stare and said, "I haven't even gotten started with the questions yet. Sammy's my child and I *have* to understand

what's going on with him." I couldn't muster a glare exactly like you used to give me, but it was pretty darn good.

I think Dr. Marris was taken aback. He rifled through his file cabinet and found me a listing of what Sammy should eat and what he should avoid. Mom, I had to ask for this!

I know we're coming down to Emporia to see you and Dad two weekends from now, so here's a list that may help you with meal planning. Well, the bad news is that your cherry Jell-O made with Coca-Cola is out. And your cherry pie. But your beef stew is in. . . . It's the best in five states.

Mom, here are the main things Sammy shouldn't eat. Dr. Marris explained to me that because the child's liver is compromised, certain substances cause the liver to become inflamed or store more glycogen. His new diet is like managing a child with type 2 diabetes, so basically, we can't let Sam's blood sugar go above 120 or below 80. Dr. Marris said something about if the blood sugar goes too low, lactic acid will build up.

Dr. Marris says that Sammy should have complex carbohydrates like whole-grain pasta or wheat bread, but only about fifteen grams per meal and five per midday snacks. I found out three saltines have five grams of carbs. Three saltines! That's not much at all to eat. The whole-grain carbs and Argo cornstarch take longer for Sammy to digest, so they release glucose more slowly. That, in turn, will give our Sammy longer periods of energy.

We started putting the Argo cornstarch in water, not milk, because I found out that milk contains sugar. Sammy and I mix up cornstarch and water in two plastic cups and make a contest of it. Who can drink the cornstarch first? Well, Mom, the mixture tastes like milk of magnesia gone bad, but I tell Sam the mixture will give us superpowers. His fingernails have even started to grow—I've never had to cut them before.

The handout also says that Sam shouldn't have lactose, fructose, or sucrose. He can also have almost any type of vegetable, but not more than one packet of ketchup with a meal. Mom, since when is ketchup a vegetable? Well, most plain meats are okay. Here's some good news. Sam can have plain popcorn, pretzels, baked corn chips, and saltines. I have a feeling that more than a bite or two of Chuck E. Cheese's pizza is going to be out. I'll have to watch everything I cook and everything Sammy snacks on, all day, every day. I think I'll make a list of approved foods to give to moms when Sammy starts to have playdates. We can do this. We *will* do this.

I must go throw in a load of laundry. Tell Dad hi and to stay off the ice cream.

Love, Janet

14

Disaster One

Cornstarch. Dr. Marris. Jumpin' Johnnie's. Tee's concert at school. Haircuts. Groceries. Laundry. Dr. Willerton. Blood work. Ultrasounds. Life rolled on, in an ultra-busy-but-smooth way, I thought, considering we were a GSD family now. Martin ping-ponged back and forth to Paris, and I had learned that being a Captain of Industry was a lot of work and, quite often, annoying. Martin hated travel and the endless waiting in airports, or the business dinners that ended at eleven o'clock at night. But we needed Martin's job, and his insurance plan was better than mine. The needle biopsies, blood work, and ultrasounds had come to thousands of dollars, but thankfully insurance paid part of the cost.

Tee came home one day from school, his pool-blue eyes watery, his freckled nose red and gooey. "My throat feels spicy, like my socks," Tee whined to me.

I spent two days at home with Tee, catching up on work

at night. Tee and I watched hours of *Looney Tunes*, sneaked in mac and cheese when Sam napped, and built gi-nor-mous Lincoln Log towers. Mostly, we rocked in my old oak rocker, reading *Frog and Toad Are Friends* and singing "Amazing Grace." Tee would hunch down on my shoulders, swiping his snotty nose periodically. When I took him in to Dr. Willerton, the pediatrician didn't find a fever or strep. It was just "one of those nasty viruses," and we had to wait it out.

On Wednesday, Tee was ready to head back to school. I knew he was feeling better, because we had the usual morning battle over clothes. I was tired and Tee won. He went to school wearing Ninja Turtle clothing in every color. Oh well, he was on the mend. We drove to school in my old powder-blue station wagon, a small pool of oatmeal jiggling in the cup holder. It had been there for five days.

That night, when I got home from work, Retha was holding Sammy. He looked limp, and his eyes were glassy.

"This little guy's not feeling well."

I could tell. Sam felt a little warm to the touch, and sure enough, the thermometer told me 101. I had been in meetings all afternoon, and Retha hadn't been able to reach me, as our department assistant had been out with the flu.

That night for dinner, I held Sam and tried to get some Gerber's bean-and-bacon toddler food into him. I had stirred in a bit of cornstarch. Nothing. Sammy was not interested, turning his head weakly to the side. "Have a bit of a saltine," I encouraged. Nope. I tried everything: a tiny bit of a hot dog. A pretzel. Even a sip or two of forbidden warm milk. Children's liquid Tylenol for the fever? Nope. I didn't know what to do.

That night I slept poorly. Dr. Marris and I had not talked about what to do if Sam got a cold or the flu. That man was pure scientist. Dr. Marris's idea of instruction was to throw the phone number for NORD at me. At any rate, I got up with my alarm at 3:00 a.m. I needed, I wanted Martin to be there. He was always the wise sage; he would know what to do. I felt so inadequate and worried about Sammy's refusal to eat or take cornstarch.

Sam was still hot; 100 now. I rocked Sam and sang to him, trying to get some warm milk and cornstarch down him. Sammy would not open his mouth.

At 6:30 a.m., I checked on Sammy.

Sammy lay on his side between two rolled baby blankets—the way the pediatrician had taught us, to prevent suffocation. I could barely see golden curls and the curve of Sammy's cheek—one hand curled near his mouth. Sammy's chest rose softly up and down.

I put my hand gently on Sam's cheek. Still warm. But what was it?

I hesitated for a second, then two, then three, hovering over the crib. Didn't it seem that he was breathing faster than normal? I racked my brain. Had I ever seen this with Tee? A gentle up down, up down, like a tiny bellows. One, two, three, four. That fast.

It was nearly 7:00 a.m. I ran to my desk and called the number on my memo pad. Dr. Marris's emergency line. I got an irritated-sounding attendant.

"Uh, hello? This is Janet Hayles. My son, Sammy, is a patient of Dr. Marris. He has glycogen storage disease. No, glycogen storage disease. Glycogen—ahhh!" The attendant, slurping coffee in the background, had no clue what I was saying. "Listen!" I said to her. "Sammy's really sick. He's breathing funny, I think—too fast. We need to come in. Yes, I'll hold. Please hurry." I paced the hallway outside Sammy's bedroom.

Ten minutes later, Retha had arrived to handle Tee's morning routine. Cornstarch bag packed, I bundled Sammy into the station wagon. Children's Mercy Hospital was a good thirty-five minutes away, through downtown traffic. As I drove, the blocks crawled by. Tick. I looked back at Sam. A breath in, a breath out. One two three four. Tick.

I carried the limp Sammy into Dr. Marris's office. He looked at Sammy for a few seconds on the exam table and barked, "Follow me!"

I scrambled down the hall after Dr. Marris with Sammy in my arms. I hadn't known the doctor could move so fast. We burst through one set of scratched gray doors. A turn. Another set of doors. Another endless hallway. Into the emergency room. Onto a gurney.

***

"I need an IV bolus of glucose—five percent glucose with point four five sodium chloride and potassium twenty milliliters. Nonlactated ringers. *Now!*" ER personnel scrambled as Dr. Marris gave orders. I backed away from the gurney. The doctors knew we had a child clinging to life.

Within seconds, one doctor had a needle in Sammy's arm, changing the needle for a small plastic tube and taping the area securely. Sam was so sick that his wails were weak, pathetic. The doctor drew vials of blood from Sammy's arm and handed them to a nurse, who scurried away to the lab. Another nurse swiftly placed a catheter from the plastic tube in Sam's arm into the nearby IV bag and Kangaroo pump. Within just a few minutes, the pump clicked, dripping life-saving glucose into the sick child.

I sat shaking two hours later in Sammy's hospital room, one arm draped over the rail of Sam's bed, touching—just touching—those baby curls. The reality smacked me: I had nearly lost my child. As Sammy drifted off to sleep with the steady click of the Kangaroo pump, I quickly ran to the nearby nurse's station and called Martin collect. It was about seven o'clock in the evening in Paris. I caught him at the hotel, and he made arrangements to catch the first flight out to Kansas City. I called Retha, and that saint—that redheaded saint—called her family and told them she would be at our home that night.

"What happened to Sammy?" I peppered Dr. Marris with questions as soon as he came into our hospital room at about ten fifteen that morning. Guilt and shame had been creeping into me like an evil fog curling, wafting. This couldn't be my baby, sick, lifeless. I had thought I had been doing GSD "right"—maybe I was just an incompetent mom?

"Sammy has metabolic lactic acidosis from the flu. When he wouldn't eat or do his cornstarch, his blood sugar dropped below normal. His body's level of ketones built up and acidified the blood, making lactic acid rise. Lactic acid should not be above seven point four, and Sammy's was above that. In other words, Sammy's blood profile had begun to crumble. Also, his liver was unable to remove the excess lactic acid. That's why he was tired and breathing so rapidly. We're running several tests every three hours on Sammy. I've requested a basic metabolic panel to check his kidney function. We're also looking at Sammy's calcium, protein, blood sugar, and electrolyte levels. We'll also catch another urine sample."[1]

"So, I should always bring Sammy into the hospital anytime he gets the flu?" I was beginning to get the picture.

"Anytime Sammy won't eat or do his cornstarch, you need to bring him in immediately. *Immediately.*" Dr. Marris paused to catch a quick breath, looking at me severely over his readers. "This goes for strep, chicken pox, high fevers, Lyme disease, or any vomiting. Sammy's body cannot fight off these conditions without having blood-sugar issues."

I wished I had known this from the get-go. I looked over

---

1. Corey Whelan, "Lactic Acidosis: What You Need to Know," Healthline, last modified March 16, 2022, https://www.healthline.com/health/lactic-acidosis.

at Sammy, who was curled in a fetal position with tubes coming out of both arms. I wanted to throw something—anything. *Why hadn't this man taught me how vulnerable Sammy was with any kind of illness? What kind of doctor was this?* I was angry—angry at fate that had given me GSD. Angry at Dr. Marris. I was especially angry at myself.

As if on cue to calm me down, a sweet-faced nurse came into the room to complete the three-hour blood sample. She paused, a kind hand on Sammy's forearm. "Well, Mr. Sammy! I'm Janice, and I'll be with you until ten o'clock tonight. Then Miss Ira comes in. We're going to get a little blood from George here. See? This little port here is called George. He takes all the sticks and the blood draws—not you! No more ouchies, okay?"

Janice tickled Sammy under the chin for a second and was rewarded by a weak smile and big blue eyes that studied her.

In the next eight days, George got stuck every three hours, day and night. IV bag solutions got changed; the Kangaroo pump clicked away. Click. Get better, Sammy. Click. Mom's here. Click. I'm so sorry, Sammy. Click. The days became a blur of faces: the doctors, the young residents with their clipboards and nervous faces, Dr. Marris's stern presence, the dietitian, the cleaners, our minister, Martin's anxious and drawn face, friends with stuffed dinosaurs and Mylar balloons. The support was overwhelming.

> And the Lord whispered, "My precious
>   child, I love you and will
> never leave you
> Never, ever, during your trials and
>   testings.
> When you saw only one set of footprints,
> It was then that I carried you."[2]

---

2. "Footprints in the Sand," Only the Bible, April 26, 2010, https://www.onlythebible.com/Poems/Footprints-in-the-Sand-Poem.html.

Sammy and I rocked in the hospital room each day, watching *Barney and Friends* and *Mister Rogers' Neighborhood* for hours. Holding his dee dee, Sammy sang along weakly to "I Love You." One day, he turned his head to me mid-rock and said, "When can Tee-Tee come give me a dee dee ride with booster jets?" Amen. Sammy was on the mend.

Meanwhile, my little world of "tackle problems like a pit bull" had crumbled. My plan A of a successful life of control was in shambles; plan B had taken off, with me chasing it breathlessly.

15

Now

When Sammy nearly died from the flu, I started reading everything I could about other children with chronic illnesses and disabilities. What had I done wrong? Did other parents live in a world of doubt, of fear, like I did—all the time?

Lubkin's Chronic Illness textbook tells me that illness "is the human experience of a disease and refers to how the disease is perceived, lived with, and responded to by individuals, their families, and health-care professionals."[1] A disability, on the other hand, is a "physical or mental condition that limits a person's movements, senses, or activities."[2] A chronic illness or disability is even more complex in character. Lubkin indicates that the chronic element incudes "permanency, residual

---

1. Pamala D. Larsen, *Lubkin's Chronic Illness* (Boston, MA: Jones and Bartlett Learning, 2019), 4.
2. "Disability," Google search, accessed February 5, 2020, https://www.google.com/search?rlz=1C5CHFA_enUS778US778&ei=NXk8XoC9K6eltgXg4rWgCg&q=definition+of+a+disability&oq.

disability, non-pathologic alteration, and required rehabilitation or a long period of supervision."[3] The text indicates that how much a person's lifestyle changes can relate to his *perceptions and beliefs* about the disease—more than the disease itself.[4] In Sammy's case, his mutated gene was in every cell of his body. No magical medicine existed to "fix" Sammy. All we could do was manage the condition—every three hours, for a total of 2,920 times per year, for as long as he lived. A slipup of six hours could mean a seizure or coma; a slipup of twelve hours, death.

I slowly plowed through memoirs of children and adults with chronic conditions after Sammy had nearly died. I intentionally picked a variety of issues: spina bifida, narcolepsy, multiple sclerosis, cerebral palsy, autism, trisomy 8 mosaicism, severe food allergies, and type 1 diabetes. What could I learn from other parents, and could I find reassurance? How did their lives compare to my experience?

My first ah-ha was that as a parent, I had tended to assume that my Sammy could or couldn't do certain things, simply because he was chronically ill. This assumption was so ironic, because a central theme of this memoir is how a parent can raise a child to be independent, given the parameters of the chronic condition.

One book I read, *Cora Means Heart*, reveals that Cora's mother struggles with the same issue of assumptions: most certainly a chronically ill child can only do so much. She writes, "Children with spina bifida see a lot of doctors."[5] Yes, they certainly do. Children or adults with spina bifida have a congenital defect of the spine. Part of the spinal cord and its meninges (membranes) are exposed through a gap in the backbone. This can cause paralysis in the lower limbs and

---

3. Larsen, *Chronic Illness*, 5.
4. Larsen, *Chronic Illness*, 4.
5. J. A. Busick, *Cora Means Heart: Memoirs of a Special Needs Mom* (CreateSpace Independent Publishing Platform, 2018), 18.

can also cause mental handicaps. Cora, like many others with this chronic condition, has a shunt or a tube in the brain. The tube tunnels under the skin with the other end of the tube ending in the abdomen, which then drains off excess cerebrospinal fluid. Unfortunately, Cora needs the shunt replaced periodically, entailing surgery. On top of that, she continues to have ultrasounds of her kidneys and bladder as well as extensive blood work to check for kidney and bladder functions. Her bladder must be drained via a catheter. Cora's condition means that she can't walk without braces and her growth hormones are low. Does this sound like a lot of medical issues? You bet.

J. A. Busick, Cora's mother, is a force of courage. She writes about her older daughter, Ashley, who began playing organized basketball at age three through the YMCA in Owensboro, Kentucky. Cora, at age three, wanted to play the sport, too, even though she had just started walking with braces and had a tube running through her body. Busick admits that Cora's basketball interest was "nowhere on my mental map of life."[6] Neither was having a disabled child.

Busick found a program in her hometown called Upward, where "every kid plays, and every kid scores."[7] Now, when I read this, I wondered, *How can a child in braces ever play basketball?* As the old expression says, "never say never" to a determined mother and a hopeful child. Busick relates that at the end of the first season of basketball, the coach put down Cora's crutches and lifted her up so she could drop the ball into the eight-foot-high basket. Busick marvels, "The crowd went wild. It was Cora's first basket."[8] The mother reveals that by the end of Cora's third year of basketball, she had taught herself to shoot one-handed into an eight-foot goal. Busick was amazed

6. Busick, *Cora Means Heart*, 30.
7. Busick, *Cora Means Heart*, 31.
8. Busick, *Cora Means Heart*, 31.

that the disabled or chronically ill kids could do things she herself couldn't do.

I didn't know this at the time, but I, too, would fall into the trap of assuming my Sammy couldn't do this or that. There came a time when Sammy was on a summer swim team with Tee. Somehow, I had volunteered as swim-team coordinator, even though I barely knew a flip turn from a dolphin kick. At that time in the 1990s, we lived in a sleepy lake community west of Kansas City called Lake Quivira. Tee was twelve and reigning king of the butterfly stroke and the breaststroke. Sam was six, still with a moderate belly. Sam would typically muster through the backstroke for one lane or two until his energy gave out.

The city kids were daunted by swimming at Lake Quivira. Our dock formed a three-sided angular C into the lake, jutting out from a sandy beach. We adults would get the ribbons ready, rope off the lanes, dig out the bullhorn, and ready the score pads. Then—most importantly—I'd get fish feed out of my backpack. Each swim meet, one swimmer got to do the honors. Plink! Plink! Plink! The kid would run around the dock, flinging the feed into the warm, murky lake. Within seconds, catfish and bluegill would swarm the waters—right before the city kids walked down the beach to the dock.

Our secret weapon for each meet was Catfish Charley. Now, Charley had been hanging around the Lake Quivira waters for three or four years at least. Charley loved two things: fish feed and nibbling on city kids' toes. At a hefty length of three feet, Charley simply unnerved our competition.

Sammy would swim the backstroke faithfully each competition. I'd walk along close to his lane and wait in angst, ready to jump in to rescue him. Stroke, gasp, sink, float up. Stroke, gasp, sink, float up. Each time, Sammy would rally to the water's surface while I readied to dive in. Somehow, he always finished the lane and got the yellow fourth-place ribbon. Sammy was determined. If Tee could swim, so could he. Why not?

At the end-of-summer championships, I drove Tee to Bonner Springs, Kansas, to compete. No Catfish Charley to help us there, but earlier that day, my son had scooped up a vial of precious Lake Quivira water. Plink! Plink! Plink! The brownish lake water splattered into the fancy Bonner Springs pool. Thus, Catfish Charley swam with us in spirit. I could just see him waving back and forth slowly, mottled, whiskers twitching, wise eyes taunting: "We're gonna get you, city kids."

Sammy was at Farmstead with Amy, our caregiver, during the final tournament, because his total season points were low—a succession of fourth-place ribbons. I knew there was no way he could compete against the jocks from Bonner, Turner, and Shawnee. No way.

"Sammy Hayles."

I had just been over to the judges' booth to check on Lake Quivira's total points.

"Sammy Hayles."

Crap. Oh, crap. The announcer was calling Sammy to compete. And Sammy was thirty miles away, oblivious, throwing feed to goats. The child could have competed—*should have competed,* and GSD wasn't the culprit here. Amy wasn't the culprit. Sammy wasn't the culprit. I was. I had assumed Sammy wouldn't compete at the championships because of his GSD and series of fourth-place ribbons. If I couldn't truly believe in him, then who would? I resolved to never—to never—*ass*ume what Sam could or couldn't do. How could he learn independence if *I* didn't truly believe in him?

Sammy's situation at the swim trials was so much like Cora's in *Cora Means Heart*. Never tell a child with GSD that he can't swim and compete. Never tell Cora, a child with spina bifida, that she can't play basketball. In all likelihood, you'll get surprised.

16

Tolerex

After Sammy's eight-day stay at Children's Mercy Hospital, life returned to normal, sort of. By this point, 1996, Sammy was nearly age four. It was time again for the bimonthly appointment with Dr. Marris.

"Hmmmm." Dr. Marris tapped Sammy's stomach, measured his legs, checked his fingernails. He gently touched Sammy's pink cheeks that had become less Gerber baby–like over the past few months.

I spun into mommy-alert-mode. What was "Hmmmm"?

Dr. Marris adjusted his glasses and looked at a recent ultrasound report. "Sammy's liver has shrunk quite a bit, which is a good thing. It means glycogen is not being stored in the liver as much and the cornstarch is doing its work. And he's walking well. Great vocabulary—do you read to him a lot? However, Sammy's growth rate—see on this chart? It's not where it should be. Here's the average for a four-year-old male.

Down here is Sammy. I recommend we have a gastrostomy tube placed into his stomach for an intake of Tolerex at night. It should be the additional nutrition Sammy needs to catch up on his growth. Children with GSD, even the males, will only grow to about five foot four, unless we take extra steps."

I had no idea what a gastrostomy tube was, or Tolerex, for that matter. *A tube in Sammy's tummy? More surgery? No!*

I calmed myself down. "Can you tell me how this works? How does the Tolerex get into Sammy's stomach at night? What is this tube you are talking about?" My gut began to do a panicked churn, an all-too-familiar feeling with me.

Dr. Marris gave me one of his looks. "Tolerex is a formula that delivers one hundred percent free amino acids, but with very few calories from fat. It's normally used with people who have a severely impaired GI function. We can use Tolerex for tube feeding or oral use. After Sammy has a gastrostomy tube placed through the abdomen and into the stomach—"

"Wait, wait!" I interrupted. "Surgery? A *hole* clear into his stomach?"

"Yes," continued Dr. Marris, seeming irked at the interruption. "Our pediatric GI surgeon will cut here." Dr. Marris touched the left side of Sammy's abdomen, across from the liver. "A temporary twelve-inch Foley will be placed in the incision. The tubing on the outside of the stomach will need to be securely taped. After the healing period is over—say three weeks—the GI surgeon will place a much simpler Foley, called a Mic-key button, in the abdomen. It lies flat to the skin's surface. It has a balloon inside the stomach keeping it in place, as well as a locking mechanism on the top, so you can twist and lock in tubing from an IV bag containing the Tolerex. You'll have a home health-care nurse show you how to operate the Kangaroo pump that meters out the Tolerex through the night. While Sammy is on nightly Tolerex, he won't need cornstarch until morning. The Tolerex will have to be special ordered at your local pharmacy."

All I could think of was *The surgeon will cut here. Clear through the stomach. A Foley hanging out. Open wound. Another surgery. More trauma for Sammy.*

Thankfully, Martin was in town for a couple of days. That night, he read stories to Tee. I could hear him declare, "Yes, I love you *this* much. *Thiiiiiis* much! *Thiiiiiiiiiiiiiiis* much!" In the other bedroom, I had selected a children's book of Bible stories for Sammy. We had just finished learning about Jacob and his coat of many colors. We had looked at pictures of Moses and the burning bush. You could say we were on a theological roll that night. I had to busy myself and be near to Sammy. It was reassuring just to touch those curls.

"Does God ever have to take a bath?" Sammy interrupted me in the midst of the burning bush story.

I was flummoxed. My spiritual background was definitely iffy. I'd been to church every Sunday my whole life, because my father was a "PK" (preacher's kid). You went to church unless you were coughing or burning with fever.

I'd always thought of God like Charlton Heston in *The Ten Commandments.* I was sure he wasn't as good-looking as Heston, of course, but thought that he would have a long gray beard and flowing robes. Perhaps stern, flashing eyes. After all, he had to do a lot of smiting in the Old Testament, and I spent a good deal of my childhood trying not to be smote. I believed in God, of course, but he was kind of like someone on the other end of a 911 call. I could get him if I needed him. Mostly, I could handle life. At least I thought so until Sammy was born.

"Uh. Well. Uh. I don't know if God even has feet." *What a lame reply, Janet.* "Maybe he's like a gentle spirit. Like a soft fog that wraps around us and loves us very much. Do you remember that day we saw fog in the woods by our house—how it curled softly around the pine trees and puffed up through the goldenrod? Actually, Sammy, I don't really know how to tell you about God. You'll feel him when he's near. I think he's almost always near." I thought back to my poem "Footprints"—those words that comforted my heart.

Sammy reflected on this, silent. I can still picture him clutching Barney and flipping his dee dee against one cheek. Our theology was good, for now. There would be many tougher questions later on.

With the kids in bed, Martin and I sat in our family room, debating about the gastrostomy tube. It would be Sammy's third surgery in three years. We didn't know what to do. All surgeries carried risks. Were we right in subjecting our child to yet another terrifying experience?

At the end of our deliberations, we decided we had to give Sammy every chance to grow—to be his best, whatever that might look like. A child with a "forever" cornstarch habit, but a child with a chance. The surgery was on.

***

The gastrostomy at Children's Mercy went smoothly. We had learned from the previous two surgeries to coordinate with the attending anesthesiologist beforehand. Sammy was allowed some light food and cornstarch the morning of the surgery. Once he was under the general anesthesia, the specialist would pump Sammy's stomach empty, switching him simultaneously to a glucose drip before and during the procedure. The drip had to stay in place for two hours after Sammy woke up until he could hold down cornstarch, water, and a light snack.

The day before the procedure, we had told Sammy he was getting a special button in his tummy for a few years—kind of like pop tabs he'd seen on the Coke cans at Grandma B.'s house. I showed Sammy a packet of Tolerex, which I special ordered from Rite Aid. It would become Sammy's fifty-six-dollar-a-week habit for some time to come. I opened a packet and let Sammy look.

"See? It's just a powder, and we'll mix it up every night in water before story time. It will go into your tummy very slowly, all night long. You'll grow and soon get as tall as Tee!"

"It stinks!"

Sammy was right. Once he was on the Tolerex regimen, I would dump a packet and sixteen ounces of water in my blender at night, watching the milky goo whirl and slop. The smell *would* knock you over; it was like rotting library paste. I typically had about thirty seconds to pour the mixture in the IV bag and scrub the blender. The Tolerex mixture would set, and I could have patched my tires with the stuff.

Sammy never knew the struggles we had with our insurance company over the Tolerex. Our first insurance claim got fired back to us like a pop fly off Derek Jeter's bat. I refiled, including two letters of medical necessity—one from our pediatrician, and one from Dr. Marris. Certainly, a letter from the head of genetics from Children's Mercy . . .

Nope. The claim was fired back. "Your insurance does not cover nutritional supplements. See paragraph seventeen, clause two."

I fired back with equal venom. "In this case, it's *not used* as a nutritional supplement. It is to help our child with GSD grow appropriately. This is GSD—a rare endocrine condition. Here is another copy of the letters of medical necessity."

Nope. A three-week period of silence from the insurance company. Another rejection. The do loop continued four more times. *What is this game?* I screamed inwardly. I wanted to find the claims reviewer and shake her until her eyes rattled.

In desperation, Martin walked in one day to the office of the vice president of Human Resources at his work. Fortunately, the two had been in meetings together before. Martin later told me what transpired.

"See these applications and letters of medical necessity? We've tried everything. Can you help us?" Martin fanned the forms out like a loaded deck of all black spades.

Sharon—the VP—had no children of her own. She was, as we say, a tough cookie in the business world; most of her co-workers were afraid she would gut them and string them up. In fact, everyone secretly called her "Attila the Hun-y." "Just a minute," she said. Sharon flipped through her Rolodex and dialed a number.

"Yes, this is a claim from Martin Hayles on behalf of child Sammy Hayles. Here's his ID number. Actually, there are six claims for Tolerex. You see them? Okay. Pay them. From now on."

That quickly, our Tolerex costs were reimbursed over the next eight years. As it turned out, Martin's company actually paid for employee benefits while the health insurance company was merely the administrator of those benefits. However, it struck me: What would it be like to raise a child with no insurance? No job? With no Martin? With no VP to turn to? The reality was that insurance and medical care worked well for those of us with connections.

Fortunately, Tolerex is covered by our government's Food Stamp Program. However, Medicaid places many restrictions on Tolerex and, more importantly, gastrostomies. According to the Finnegan medical supply website, "Insurance will only cover feeding tubes if the patient is 100 percent tube fed for all nutrition and liquids. This means that you can never feed the patient by mouth. If a DME [durable medical equipment] company is told a patient can take even a spoonful of liquid orally, they legally cannot provide the feeding tube, and all the materials will have to be paid for out of pocket."[1] Tolerex,

1. SuLauren Wilson, "What Is a Feeding Tube, and How Do I Get Insurance

Kangaroo pumps, and home health-care nurses are expensive. What about a chronically ill child whose parents don't have insurance? He doesn't get the proper care.

***

The harsh truth is that not all parents with special needs children are lucky enough to have jobs or insurance. *Waking Mathilda*, one of the books I had read after Sammy's close call, illustrates just this point. The author, Claire Crisp, was a physical therapist in London, with three children and a husband who was a professor. When the H1N1 pandemic of 2009 hit, Crisp had her daughter Mathilda vaccinated with squalene, according to the British government's recommendations. The seemingly innocuous, five-second vaccination went awry. Crisp found out later that this vaccine had been tested only on a small portion of adults and on no children. Within weeks, Mathilda began having nighttime hallucinations. She would sometimes collapse during the day, folding in half at the waist and falling to the floor. She began to turn quiet, introverted. She slept during the day, waking up for minutes, only to fall asleep again. She developed ataxia, or muscle weakness of the legs and speech organs. After two years of doctors and tests, Mathilda was diagnosed at age three as the youngest patient in history with narcolepsy.

Waking Mathilda focuses on the sheer monumental task of a mom and dad raising a child who sleeps, collapses, and hallucinates twenty-four hours a day. The parents must care for their two other healthy children at the same time—and money is tight. Oliver, the father, is a college professor struggling to stay employed. Crisp writes about the year 2005, when

---

to Pay for One?" Finnegan Medical Supply, September 2, 2014, https://finneganmedicalsupply.com/blogs/news/what-is-a-feeding-tube-and-how-do-i-get-insurance-to-pay-for-one.

Oliver was between teaching jobs: "Despite the string of qualifications, degrees, publications, and professional experience, we were both officially unemployed, disillusioned, and broke. Were it not for my parents owning a tiny and spectacularly cute Victorian cottage in the heart of the New Forest, we would also have found ourselves homeless."[2] The family literally scoured the nearby forest for firewood to heat their home and for fruit for the kids. The milkman dropped off milk for the kids but always managed to throw in a loaf of bread. To compound the injury in this dilemma, the couple had previously been at Notre Dame for two years, and thus were rejected for unemployment benefits in the UK because they had been absent from the country for a year. Imagine. Two healthy kids and a third who was tremendously ill. No fallback. No money.

The narrative is every parent's nightmare as Claire and Oliver work for months to get a diagnosis for Mathilda. Finally, obtaining a diagnosis, the parents pushed physicians in order to get approval for an experimental drug known as Xyrem, compounded only in one pharmacy in Missouri and costing a resounding $3,000 per bottle. Xyrem is also known as sodium oxybate—a highly controversial drug notoriously abused as a date-rape drug with a huge street value. At Bristol Royal Hospital for Children, one of many sources Claire uncovered, she pushed Dr. Jensen for Xyrem. His response was ambivalent: "I would have to look into it. It's a very expensive drug and difficult to get a hold of. . . . We would need to make an application to the board and justify why the National Health Service should spend thousands of pounds when Xyrem isn't proven to help children as young as Mathilda. Then they will argue that for everyone like Mathilda, the same amount of money could treat, say, five other children who also need specialized

2. Claire Crisp, *Waking Mathilda: A Memoir of Childhood Narcolepsy* (USA: Palace Gates Press, 2017), 19.

medication."[3] Two months later, in despair, Claire pressed Dr. Jensen again at an office visit. She remembers the doctor reminding her that "A year's supply would cost our local health authority twelve thousand pounds."[4]

In the midst of the NHS red tape, Mathilda was fading before her parents' eyes.

In a final attempt to get help for Mathilda, the Crisp family moved to the United States near Stanford University. Oliver was fortunate to secure a teaching assignment at Stanford, and thus, incredible medical insurance became available. Had he not been employed, Mathilda's medical options would have been slim to none. Through Dr. Emmanuel Mignot, professor of sleep medicine at Stanford, the family finally got a prescription for Xyrem.

Waking Mathilda has a proverbial happy ending. Mathilda finally receives management for narcolepsy, and Oliver, the father, still teaches at a prestigious university with a robust insurance program. However, everyone is not so lucky. In fact, most of the world's population isn't.

As I think back on my son's numerous appointments, tests, scans, surgeries, and ER visits, I remember the horrible stress of *What is it? What if?* The Hayles family paid plenty of money out of pocket to help Sammy. However, we had the benefit of jobs—good jobs—and insurance. What must it have been like for Claire and Oliver Crisp to have medical uncertainty heaped on top of financial issues and government red tape? Here is my takeaway: Most parents work really hard to care for their chronically ill children. Most parents love their chronically ill children. However, what makes a big difference between a *thriving* Sammy Hayles and a child *dying* in inner city Chicago is money, insurance, and great health care. That's it.

---

3. Crisp, *Waking Mathilda*, 172.
4. Crisp, *Waking Mathilda*, 214.

***

I think back to the nights in ER at Children's Mercy whenever Sammy had a bad cold or a sore throat. We would wait in the 3:00 a.m. haze of despair. However, numerous children in that same waiting room—mostly Black—needed to see a doctor too. Any doctor. These were kids with fevers and vomiting episodes. They were waiting because no other hospital would take them. They didn't have pediatricians. They didn't get well checks. They didn't get vaccinations. The kids and parents waited, because they were part of a faceless group in the US. That faceless group is the uninsured. The uninsured leave the ER with a huge bill; their only "comfort" is that they can pay it in installments—for months.

What happens to chronically ill children when Mom and Dad don't have jobs or insurance?

In 2010, the Affordable Care Act was signed into law, putting in place comprehensive health insurance reforms that would come into effect over the next four years and beyond, with full implementation occurring on January 1, 2014. Along with this were Medicaid expansion on a state-by-state basis as well as the establishment of health insurance marketplaces. However, in 2018, "27.9 million nonelderly individuals were uninsured, an increase of nearly 500,000 from 2017."[5] According to KFF.org, most of our uninsured are low-income families with at least one worker. In fact, in 2018, 70 percent of nonelderly uninsured individuals worked for an employer that did not offer them health benefits.[6] Additionally, many of the uninsured are Black—half of the nonelderly uninsured population. The website also reports that individuals with income 200 percent below the Federal Poverty Level are at the

5. Jennifer Tolbert, Kendal Orgera, and Anthony Damico, "Key Facts about the Uninsured Population," KFF, November 6, 2020, https://www.kff.org/uninsured/issue-brief/key-facts-about-the-uninsured-population.
6. Tolbert, Orgera, and Damico, "Key Facts."

highest risk of being uninsured. In 2018, eight in ten of the uninsured were families with incomes 400 percent below the poverty level.[7]

Why on earth would people *not* get insurance? Pretty straightforward, really. According to KFF.org, "in 2018, 45 percent of uninsured adults said that they remained uninsured because the cost of coverage was too high."[8] Many jobs don't provide insurance coverage, and sadly, some poor adults live in states where Medicaid coverage has not been expanded. They get the double whammy: poverty, but not enough poverty to qualify. Additionally, it's quite common for the poor to not even know where to turn for help. And if you're an undocumented immigrant—forget it. You can't apply for Medicaid. You try to pay for your bills with cash as you get it. Mostly, you try to stay under the radar and away from Immigration and Customs Enforcement.[9]

Like the children sitting in Children's Mercy ER in Kansas City, one in five uninsured adults goes without needed medical care, according to a 2018 study.[10] Those uninsured, if they can even get to health care at a hospital, normally pay higher rates than do the insured patients. KFF.org documents that, as a result, "uninsured people are less likely than those with insurance to receive preventive care and services for major health conditions and chronic diseases."[11] Lack of outpatient care then results in hospitalizations for normally avoidable health conditions. Quite often, being poor and/or uninsured simply means imminent death. A mother doesn't bleed less for the death of a child simply because she's poor.

***

7. Tolbert, Orgera, and Damico, "Key Facts."
8. Tolbert, Orgera, and Damico, "Key Facts."
9. Tolbert, Orgera, and Damico, "Key Facts."
10. Tolbert, Orgera, and Damico, "Key Facts."
11. Tolbert, Orgera, and Damico, "Key Facts."

I had never been good at working with equipment. Even when I would use a screwdriver on a pesky cabinet door, I always used the mantra, "Lefty loosey, righty tighty." So, I was relieved the day the home health-care nurse arrived with a shiny new Kangaroo pump, IV bags, tubing, an extra Mic-key button kit, medical tape, and assorted syringes. Not to mention a travel-sized Kangaroo pump backpack. I eyed the array of equipment with anxiety.

Retha and I trained with the home health-care nurse; I worked with Martin and Tee later that evening. The Mic-key button and Tolerex became a nighttime routine. Quite often, Sammy would flip and thrash around in the night. The IV line would crimp, causing a piercing alarm that made Martin and me sprint to Sammy's room. Sometimes, the securely taped Mic-key button would unlock from the IV tubing. Oblivious, the Kangaroo pump would continue its click, click, click. We'd awaken to Sammy's howls as the sticky Tolerex ran over his pj's and the sheets, pooling onto the floor. On other occasions, about every two months, the inner balloon of the Mic-key would deflate. Out it would slip, so Martin and I would fly into Sammy's room to give him an emergency dose of cornstarch, because the Tolerex could not get into the stomach with a defective Mic-key. We'd tape the Mic-key back into Sammy's stomach, pack extra cornstarch, bundle up a sleepy Sammy and Tee, and drive to Children's Mercy ER. It was Murphy's law that the Mic-key always broke at 3:00 a.m. on a twenty-degree Kansas City night as the stars crackled in the sky. The four of us would get back home at 5:30 a.m., just in time for Martin and me to shower and head off to work. Retha would come and let Tee sleep in for the morning, his face pale from the 3:00 a.m. scramble.

After about our fourth middle-of-the-night family sojourn to ER, I decided to consult with Dr. David Roberts, a pediatric gastroenterologist at Children's Mercy. We had to do something about the frequent races to the hospital.

Dr. Roberts looked like Robert Redford—just in his early forties. With his boyish haircut and blue eyes, he also seemed like the guy next door.

"See, Sammy? Here's a new Mic-key button for you. Since you've been growing so well, we're going to go up a size. The new button has a stem that is a little longer. And see here? This is the balloon at the end of the stem that will hold it in your stomach."

"It doesn't look like a balloon," Sammy countered.

"Well, I'm going to show you how to put the new Mic-key in and then blow up the balloon. It's kind of like magic. Okay . . . first, we always wash our hands with soap and water. We sing 'Happy Birthday to You' so we know we've washed long enough."

Sammy, Dr. Roberts, and I sang enthusiastically. Dr. Roberts was most energetically off pitch the entire time, but no matter. A couple of nurses peeked in, smiling, charts in hand. "Now, Sammy, let's stand here by the exam table and gently pull out the old button. You *gently* pull. See? It comes right out, because the balloon on the end has collapsed. Now, we're going to put a bit of lubricant on the tip of the new button. It will go into your stomach slick as a whistle. Then, we'll push the Mic-key in until the pop-top is right up against your skin. Do it gently. Don't worry; your little stomach hole is all healed up."

Sammy was nearly five at this time. The world was pretty straightforward. If Dr. Roberts said to gently push the Mic-key in the hole, then that's what you did.

"Now, we have a bowl of distilled water here on the exam table. Take the little syringe that came in your Mic-key kit. Pull it apart and dip this end in the water. Good! You've filled the syringe up most of the way. Now, we're going to put eight millimeters of water in the syringe. See the marking on the syringe? This is when Mom can help you. Perfect!" Dr. Roberts continued to coach Sammy, step by step.

In a minute, Sammy surveyed his new Mic-key with interest. It lay flat and perfect against his skin.

"So how come *you* had to go to school *for so long*?" Sammy questioned Dr. Roberts.

The doctor's blue eyes crinkled with amusement. Thank goodness he thought Sammy's comment was funny.

"Well, a few things I do are harder than this, Mr. Sammy. You did a great job! Maybe medicine will be in your future."

From then on, Sammy was the master of all things Mic-key. He could change out his old button to a new one in about five minutes.

17

Academia

"I think Sammy is bored." Retha and I were having one of our end-of-workday briefings.

"I know I'm talking myself out of a job, but I think Sammy needs to go to school. We go to story time at the library, see kiddie movies, and enjoy the petting zoo in Lenexa, but it's not enough. When Tee does his homework after school, Sammy gets his pencil and does 'math' too. He's trying to teach Barney how to read. He's Mr. Social. He needs other kids around."

Retha was always right.

Tee's school was half an hour away from home but very close to my work. He had been in school since age four, too, and loved it—despite nightmare encounters with science fair projects. I still cringed when I thought of our project last month—a platform made with Popsicle sticks that had to hold ten pounds. Well, *ours didn't.* Tee had also bitten his kindergarten teacher, Mrs. Parker, three years ago. But only once and it wasn't very deep. At any rate, Martin and I made an appointment the next week to meet with the Early Years and Pre-K teachers after school.

"I recommend that Sammy start in the Early Years program, even though he could handle the cognitive activities in Pre-K," stated Mrs. Miller, a dark-haired sunbeam of a woman. I still remember Sammy wandering over to the Book Nook corner and then over to miniature easels lined with little tubs of tempera paint, just waiting to be artistically spread. And the back of the classroom—it was magnificent! Sliding red numbers in slots. A huge clock with movable hands. Blue and green bean bags and storybooks lying nearby.

I was sold; I wanted to go to Early Years myself.

When Martin and I got the kids to bed that night, my fretting started. School meant Sammy leaving his safe cocoon of family and Retha. I had to make sure that Mrs. Miller and the school nurse understood Sammy's condition perfectly. Thank goodness that I worked only five minutes from school, should something happen. I made a mental note: *Keep my cell phone with me at all times.* Our department assistant loved to take lengthy smoke breaks.

That Saturday, Sammy went down for his nap, because even a normal day tired him. I went to work, planning. I scribbled *To-Dos for School*:

- Description of GSD 1a—simple but accurate.
- How to mix up cornstarch and administer. Use large syringe into Mic-key for cornstarch—like at home?
- Need schedule for dosing. Must find out snack times and lunch at school. When is PE?
- Emergency contacts.
- Supplies: fresh boxes of Argo monthly, plastic containers, large syringes, tubing for the Mic-key, sugar-free Citrucel, anti-nausea pills, glucose gel.

- Have supplies in the classroom *and* the nurse's office?
- Keep extra supplies in my car?
- List of foods for Sammy to avoid. How to handle birthday parties?
- Low-blood-sugar warning signs written out.
- Buy string pack to hold all of Sammy's supplies.

I set my Pentel mechanical pencil down and rubbed my head. I thought I had my to-do list. I set about creating forms on my computer. Thank goodness I had gotten some helpful pages from NORD. I left voice mails with Mrs. Miller and the school nurse. I hoped I could document and communicate well so Sammy's school day would go smoothly. It was step one for a healthier childhood. How independent could Sammy ever be? I didn't have a clue, but school was a big step forward.

***

> Dear Mom,
>
> I know you are worried about little Sammy starting school so young. But I know that you as a professor love education, and I think Sammy will too. Remember—you were finished with your master's and out teaching in western Kansas by age twenty-two. Well, I think Sammy has your brains. Just the other day, I was asking the boys to pick up their toys before bedtime. Well, Tee was popping his Legos into the toy tub—he's an obedient kid unless it comes to his socks. But Sammy, good grief. Here's how the conversation went, give or take.

"I don't need to put my blocks up. I'm going to use them tomorrow. It's unnecessary." *Unnecessary?*

"Mama, I'm pretty sure you got all these toys out, so you should pick them up."

"Dad can do it. What has he done all day?" I looked over at Martin, sprawled out on the couch, *Time* magazine open, eyes closed. "Pfoooo. Pbubbbba. Pfoooo." Martin was out cold.

Mom, I just stood there during this conversation, speechless. Finally, I fell back on every parent's convenient mantra: "Because I told you so."

Well, sad news. We're going to lose Retha, because she needs to work full-time. She's like a sister and a freckled wise sage, all rolled into one. I did talk to Carol Morrison at church. She knows a young girl finishing up her elementary education degree. Anyway, her name is Amy, and she has one year left of college. She wants to work part-time, so I'll have her come over and chat with me. When both boys are in school, we'll need someone to pick them up and do snacks and homework.

Back to the school issue. I called NORD last week, and one of the staff members faxed more articles to Martin's office. So, here are some snippets I found. Can you read them to Dad too? I know he's worried about Sammy. Here's the first:

"In many ways school is a microcosm of society in general, and, in interacting with teachers and pupils, the child with a chronic illness will learn how to present their illness outside school and experience how their condition is perceived by others. Common to the majority of children with chronic illness is the desire to be treated the same as their friends."[1]

Mom, we don't know how far Sammy can progress, but I just want him to do what other kids do. Well, do whatever *he* can. Oh here: I just found two more entries:

"Every child needs to feel part of their school community. They need to take part in sports, school fundraising, drama productions and school trips."[2] I guess we'll figure how Sammy can manage these when we get to that point. It makes my head hurt to think about managing all this.

"Written information, detailing how the child is affected by their illness, the use of medication or treatment and symptoms to be watchful for, should be made available to the principal and then disseminated around the key staff members in contact with the child."[3]

You know, Mom, as I just wrote this down, I realized that I need to get all the medical information to Sammy's PE teacher too. He'll need to understand that Sammy can't handle long stretches of physical play. He'll need to understand what Sammy means when he says, "I'm cornstarch tired." And speaking of cornstarch tired, I'm tired too! Bye for now and with hugs,

Janet

---

1. This information is derived from Sharon Dempsey, *Extreme Parenting* (Great Britain: Athenaeum Press, 2008), 129.
2. Dempsey, *Extreme Parenting*, 130.
3. Dempsey, *Extreme Parenting*, 130.

18

The Big Day

I was anxious that morning. Very anxious. Could Sammy "do" school?

The blue station wagon was packed to the gills. Tee had his backpack and a huge black trash bag. Each kid had to bring one hundred objects to school and teach the other kids division problems using the objects. Tee had chosen one hundred red cups. Not something small, of course, like pennies. One hundred large Solo cups. We had practiced division the night before, lining up twenty cups here and ten over there. "See? Ten cups go into twenty"—(slide slide)—"like this. How many times did we do that?"

Tee was a whiz at reading and PE, but math was mysterious.

"Two! Three! Two and a half!" Tee shot out answers, hoping to hit the target, any ole target.

Sammy was strapped in behind me in the car. He had a new backpack—Barney, of course. It was chock-full of extra clothing, underwear, and approved GSD snacks. The string pack was inside, also, with premeasured containers of dry cornstarch, Level Life glucose gel, a large catheter tip syringe, and tubing. We had been giving Sammy's cornstarch to him through the Mic-key button, because the starch was like drinking chalk. And Sammy was so slooooowwwww.

I had been up since 5:15 a.m., fortifying myself with two hits of coffee, showering, applying makeup, and selecting a suit for the day. I was wired up, and not just from the Folgers kick. It was Sammy's sixth day of school. On top of that milestone, I had a big presentation coming up regarding the company stock plan. *Yes, okay, Janet, this suit.* A black-and-red plaid pleated midi skirt with a black boiled-wool jacket. A turtleneck. One gold chain. Earrings. My black Timex. Dark pantyhose. Demure black flats. The corporate look was complete. Watch out, world. Motherhood and the corporate world. Yeah, watch out.

Martin would usually get breakfast ready for the kids at seven. I'd flip two English muffins out of the toaster, slap on some butter, and cram my gourmet breakfast into foil. At 7:15, we'd load the car: two kids, two backpacks, one hundred Solo cups, my breakfast, and my gym bag. Mission Control: ready for departure.

The school schedule had gone swimmingly, I felt. *I've got this.*

Sammy's IV line had crimped twice during the night, sending me out of a deep sleep into a sprint down the hall to his room. Martin was in Paris that week. The middle-of-the-night chaos created bathroom trips, two rounds of "Amazing Grace," and a looooooooong back rub. The next morning, I was bleary-eyed. Despite my two cups of morning courage, I forgot to put an extra outfit and underwear in Sam's backpack.

We pulled up to the front of campus that morning. Tee hopped out with his backpack, one hundred Solo cups, and a huge rolled-up diagram that we had helped him with last night. It was sort of, kind of, a little bit like, wanted to be, could have been—a depiction of a double helix. Good grief. Why couldn't the kid ever get to do something simpler, like a chart on *Our Friend the Atom*? As Tee burst in the front door of his building, we circled to the back of the campus. I parked in front of the Early Years building and walked around to the back seat to help Sam.

There it was, simply everywhere. Apparently, something had disagreed with Sammy, and that disagreement, brown and sticky, had oozed onto Sammy's clothes, squishing onto the car seat in all directions. This was not a simple Wet Ones cleanup. As our family often phrased it, this was "a four-star poo parade."

I made a quick phone call to work, wheeling the wagon around toward home. Thirty minutes later, I carried a towel-wrapped Sammy into the huge laundry sink in our home. I stood him up, peeling layers of brown sticky clothing off him, dropping them into a bucket filled with Spic and Span suds and warm water. Sprayer and soap in hand, I tackled Sammy's tummy, legs, feet, arms, hands. Sonnie, our usually cheerful golden retriever, trotted into the laundry room and whirled back around, ears back. Wait. How did the brown disaster get behind Sam's left ear?

Back in the car. A clean Sammy. A car seat that smelled like Lysol. Thirty minutes later, we retraced our steps to the Early Years building. Sammy joined in with art time, immediately forgetting the morning mess in the excitement of tempera paint and the chance to be Jackson Pollock. I got to my office fifteen minutes later, opening up my Franklin Planner to assess the day's agenda. A shaky breath. Okay. Meeting with programmers in fifteen minutes. Employee review at one o'clock. Oh no. It was the lady who was always in a huff with me. The chip on her shoulder was the size of Texas. A stock plan update with twenty department heads.

I slammed my planner shut and took a swig of yesterday's cold coffee, the creamer skimming the surface like pale white moss. And there—*there it was*—on the cuff of my suit coat. A lovely, large brown reminder of the morning. Ground deep into the fibers and there to stay.

Did I still think I had life under control?

19

The Dice Rolls

Weekends were the best, as life slowed down by ten ticks.

On Saturday mornings, I'd grab a huge mug of coffee and milk, and both boys would sit with me on the carpet, nestled inside my legs. "Birdie in the nest," the boys would call it. We'd watch our favorite cartoons: *Scooby-Doo, The Jetsons,* and, of course, *Teenage Mutant Ninja Turtles.* Mid–turtle adventures, Tee would hop up and yell, "Turtle Power!" That was my cue to grab cup number two and rebuild our nest. Mother bird was happy and in her element.

Saturday afternoons were playtime for the kids. I remember one day in particular. It was autumn in all its Kansas perfection. The tang of smoke circling from my neighbor's leaf pile. Warm sunshine pulling dry muskiness from the earth. It was a day where nothing bad could happen.

I puttered around the cool house in my jeans and fuzzy Kansas sweatshirt. I folded dingy dish towels and tossed Legos into a cracked red toy bin. Peace. Quiet. Contentment in my heart. Tee, his friend Scott, and Sonnie galloped across our front yard and into the woods next door. A crumbling house foundation—a cool fort—enticed the three into the dense woods. Sammy, clearly reveling in his five-year-old glory, trotted slowly after the big boys. His blond curls bounced with every step.

I circled to the front door and yelled at Tee. "Hey! Make sure you take Sam with you, okay? Watch him."

"Sure, Mom." Tee's freckled, lanky arms flashed as he zoomed through patches of sun and into the treasures of the woods.

I wandered into the kitchen and began frying up hamburger, onions, and garlic. Spaghetti. My mouth watered as I tasted my batch. Humming a few bars of "A Bushel and a Peck," I wiped my oniony hands across my apron. The apron was my favorite—white, with red piping and rickrack. "Kiss the Cook!" it advertised across the front.

In twenty minutes, footsteps thumped across the back deck. Tee, Scott, and Sonnie burst into the house. Tee dumped his treasures on the Formica countertop: an old transistor radio, four bolts, and a rumpled paperback with a buxom blonde on the cover. Tee was only eleven, and I hoped he had grabbed the book out of pure curiosity.

"Mom—we're starving! Can Scott stay for dinner?" Scott, one of six kids next door, sniffed the simmering spaghetti sauce and looked at me expectantly. In his household, anything beyond mac and cheese was gourmet.

"Sure." I flicked on a light switch to inspect my hamburger concoction. I poured grains of salt into the crook of my hand, letting them flit into the spaghetti sauce. "Tee, where's your brother?"

"Don't know." Tee picked through his treasures, eyeing the buxom blonde on the book cover. The woman sure didn't look like Mom. "Well, we were exploring the woods and got hungry. I thought Sammy was following us."

A tickle of fear feathered in my gut. Sammy needed his cornstarch in about an hour.

I trotted out of the house and into the network of trees, now fading gently to blues and grays. Hidden dark pockets. Leafy dampness.

"Sam!" I called.

No answer.

Tick.

In fifty minutes, Sam's blood sugar would begin to drop. And drop. And drop—to thirty, when he would start to have seizures or lose consciousness.

Running now, I sped back to the house. "Tommy! Scott! Find Dad and start looking for Sam, *now!"*

I dashed down through my backyard, into the woods, and then down to the shore of a calm, blue lake. Water. A blue lure. Would Sammy understand? I began praying with an intensity I had never known. *Not this, God. Not this. Not Sammy.*

Forty minutes left. No Sammy. The silence screamed at me.

My husband sped down our street in the dusty blue Volvo station wagon as Sam's empty car seat straps flapped in the wind. His new favorite toy, Penny the Panda, tipped sadly in the back seat. Meanwhile, I ran back up to the house and called the Lake Quivira fire department. Sirens soon began to wail. Police cars cruised the lake perimeters. Patrol lights revolved, piercing and slicing the darkening woods.

Tick.

I raced across the street, yelling to Debbie, my neighbor, for help. She hopped on her old golf cart and roared down the street and into the green velvet of the nearby golf course.

Tick.

Fear circled my stomach, pushing its black tendrils into

my heart. I prayed again. *Not this, God. Not this. Help me. I'll do anything for you.*

I ran back into the woods—circling, circling, asking God for the crunch of footsteps or a flash of blond curls. I grabbed a tree trunk, gasping for air, listening. Faint yelling echoed across the woods.

"Janet! Janet!"

I sprinted into my front yard. What if? Sweat broke out; I smelled my fear.

I heard Debbie's cart come to a painful, dieseling halt. There she sat. And there . . . there was Sam with chocolate on his Gerber-baby face and an empty wrapper in his fist.

I ran up, grabbing Sammy, sobbing, thanking God.

"Sam! Don't ever do that again! We didn't know where you were."

"It's okay, Mama," Sam replied matter-of-factly. "I didn't know where I was either."

Mother meltdown. Relief, tears, joy, anger, guilt.

Stamped into my primal gut now is the preciousness of life. The dice rolled one time, and Sam wandered off. Roll two—he could have collapsed in the woods, sliding into shock. Roll three—he could have wandered into the lake. Roll four—my neighbor just happened to find him in the middle of a golf course, eating a Hershey bar.

I remember Tee running up to the scene, his jacket half off, his eyes panicked.

"Tee. I asked you to do one thing. And you and Scott got busy in your stupid fort and forgot about Sammy. He could have died!" The words flew out of my mouth, cruel, hurtful, as Tee's eyes turned a watery blue.

Life can flip in a minute. Had I allowed Sam too much independence at age five? Was it fair for me to burden Tee with the task of watching his little brother—again?

20

Shadow Child

Tee was a "shadow child." What a perfect name for a child who lives as a second-class citizen because of a sibling's chronic illness or disability.

I recently read about Randall S. Beach, who is a practicing attorney now. Growing up, he was the big brother to Jon, who had been diagnosed with type 1 diabetes. Beach's book, *Shadow Child,* hits frighteningly close to home in describing the life of a sibling who grows up second fiddle to the ill brother.

Randall writes of the time Jon was first diagnosed with type 1. Jon was in the hospital for a few days getting the condition under control. Randall states, "I needed to know that Jon still existed and was going to come back home. It had only been a few days, but to my seven-year-old mind, those days had been weeks . . . being without a mom was worse. Grandma and Auntie always made sure I was taken care of and fed well

. . . but they were not adequate substitutes for Mom. I needed my mom. I wanted her back."[1] I think about Randall's reaction to Jon's hospital visit. Ironically, my two children were about the same age when Sammy spent days at Children's Mercy. My husband managed to juggle work and hospital visits, pulling in his mother for help and stringing together hot dog meals for Tee. Tee's homework and sporting events went on the back burner, as did the nighttime stories.

The sibling of a chronically ill child not only misses his parents, but he also sees the ill child getting "special" treatment. Beach writes that he was a bit jealous of Jon's novelty dinners in bed in the hospital. He remembers: "It seemed that my brother was having a pretty good time in the hospital."[2] In like manner, this is what our son Tee probably saw. Sammy's time in Children's Mercy meant multiple staff visitors, Mylar balloons, and meals in bed. It meant Mom rocking him for hours. It meant all the cartoons he could handle. Meanwhile, Tee got hot dogs, school, a missing mom, and homework.

Beach also describes his feelings when he was brought into Jon's care routine—much against his will. On occasions, Jon's blood sugar would drop, or he'd have a spike after an insulin injection. One time, the family was heading back from the Boston Museum of Science when Jon began screaming and shaking in the back of the car. Speeding down the Mass Pike at sixty miles an hour, Beach's mother handed big brother a wad of honey packets from the glove box. Beach hopped in the back seat. He recalled: "I pressed my body against my brother's jerking movements and tore open the first honey packet. When Jon's mouth opened with a scream, I thrust the packet into the side of his mouth and squeezed. . . . His jaw clamped tight, and a small gurgle came from somewhere; then it opened again with another scream. All at once, through slits in my brother's

1. Randall S. Beach, *Shadow Child* (USA: Outskirts Press, 2017), 39.
2. Beach, *Shadow Child*, 43.

eyes, I saw his eyeballs roll back into his head. He was having a seizure."[3] Fortunately, Mom was close to Camp Joslin, a special diabetes summer camp that Jon was attending. She wheeled the car into the camp, where doctors got Jon into the infirmary and stabilized him. Within an hour, Jon was back to normal and trotted off, laughing with a camp counselor, to enjoy archery. Meanwhile, Beach sat on the porch of the main camp building, sobbing from the rawness of the afternoon. He had been traumatized by being so close to a life-and-death situation. He recalls: "My most important job was to take care of my brother. . . . No matter what happened to me, I was to be thankful that I was spared the disease borne by Jon."[4] In a similar manner, our son Tee was often too involved in Sammy's emergencies. Tee was dragged to the ER many nights when Sammy was vomiting or needed a new Foley. Tee was privy to all the midnight Kangaroo pump alarms and Sammy's wails if his blood sugar dipped.

Beach makes another important point about being a shadow child. He states, "From my perspective, my baby brother fast became my babied brother in many ways. Jon's well-being became my mother's number one priority, and his happiness became her second. . . . I am confident that my mother wished the same for me then and does to this day. The difference was that she had to be actively engaged in the management of my brother's health and in doing so, became actively engaged in the management of his happiness."[5] As I read Beach's words, I thought, *Convicted!* Martin and I tried our best to divide our time between Tee and Sammy. However, GSD is a jealous and demanding mistress. When Sammy would have a blood-sugar episode, all attention flew his way. End of story.

Beach indicates that, for all the reasons described above,

---

3. Beach, *Shadow Child*, 59.
4. Beach, *Shadow Child*, 65.
5. Beach, *Shadow Child*, 75.

jealousy entered into his relationship with Jon. He recalls one particular incident involving a log cabin.

Jon and Randall had a crude lean-to out in the woods near their home—much like the fort Tee and Sammy loved to play in as children. Over time, Jon began to take an interest in log cabins, so his parents decided he should have a real one. This project involved clearing the woods, pouring a concrete slab, and building a two-story structure, complete with four working glass windows, an asphalt roof, and a door. It was essentially Jon's cabin, and pretty darn nice.

Interesting, I thought as I read about the cabin. *This sounds like the time we bought a shed for Sammy.*

When Sammy was about seven, he, too, longed for a "real" fort or playhouse. Oh yes—he also wanted a trampoline.

"You would always know where we were, Mom," Sam would argue. "We wouldn't track mud into the house. We could play in the shed. We could nurture our creativity." *Nurture our creativity?* Oh brother. He was a marketing man already—all he needed was some snake oil, a platform, and a tent.

The arguments would continue nonstop. "The trampoline would be a cool place for all my friends to hang." "Think of the exercise!" "You don't want me playing video games, do you?" "We could put our bicycles in the shed. It would give you more room in the garage." Sammy would inhale deeply and blast me for another fifteen minutes nonstop. *Nonstop.*

What Sharon Dempsey writes in *Extreme Parenting* is true. As she describes, "It is all too common to try to overcompensate for the child's health problems. Many parents find that they want to give their child everything to somehow make up for the deficit that fate appears to have bestowed."[6] Had Dempsey been watching the Hayles family through a figurative window? Much like the journalist described in her book, Martin and I finally caved in to Sammy and bought a $1,000

6. Dempsey, *Extreme Parenting,* 1.

assembled shed. With cute white siding and black shutters, it was every kid's dream. Additionally, a trampoline arrived, becoming the social center of the neighborhood. Both boys were living the dream, except this was really all to make Sammy happy. And Tee knew it.

Did Tee act out because he became the "shadow child"? Of course.

When Sammy was in grade school and Tee was in high school, Tee's favorite trick involved waiting until Sammy was in the shower. Tee would head into our backyard on a hot summer afternoon, where cicadas perched, chirping on our trees. Tee would scoop up his buggy friends, sneak into the bathroom, and dump twenty flailing cicadas on Sammy's head. You could hear the screams for miles. Occasionally, Tee would keep his pranks simpler. Once, he put a bit of Ex-Lax in Sammy's almond milk. Many bathroom visits later, Sammy determined the culprit. Another time, Tee sneaked into the bathroom, again, during Sammy's shower. This time, he sprayed voluminous clouds of Lysol disinfectant into the air, running out and holding the bathroom door shut. Sammy's screams brought Martin and me running to the rescue. Minutes later, the two boys sat in separate time-outs, Sammy sulky and angry—Tee rather smug at the apparent leveling of justice.

***

Dear Tee,

Here you are a six-foot grown man, but you're still Tee to me. You always will be.

I just have to write that I'm sorry. I'm sorry for all the times you got dragged to the ER because Sammy's Mic-key button came out or he started vomiting. I'm sorry for the eight days I was in the hospital with Sammy and the nurses wouldn't let you come visit. Sammy got balloons and you got hot dogs at home. Plus, you needed your mom. I'm sorry that I burdened you with Sammy's care. It wasn't fair for me to teach you about giving Sammy cornstarch or how to operate the Kangaroo pump. You never really got to be a kid; you were like the third parent. I also think about the time Sammy got lost and we found him in the middle of the golf course. I think I said some hurtful things to you when you arrived at the scene, just smearing guilt on you. I remember how I yelled at you and how your blue eyes filled with guilty tears.

I'm also sorry about the time you were all excited about getting our first dog. Remember? We were going to name him Oscar. We had stopped first at McDonald's and had fun in the playscape outside. It was so strange that Sammy's sweaty leg twisted when he went down the slide, cracking his fibula. I think the ER called it a greenstick fracture, and one doctor gave me the third degree about child abuse. Sammy ended up with a bright blue cast from his groin down to his toes, and everyone fussed over him incredibly for weeks. You just took it. You wanted a dog, but you got a trip to the hospital instead.

Dad and I did our best. We tried to get to all your track events, your plays, your concerts. But, looking back on all this, I know you sometimes got the shaft. It wasn't fair that your needs sometimes got shoved aside because I had to run to the hospital with Sammy or pick up more Tolerex—or, or, or.

I look at you now—what a man you are! An A student with a business degree and an MBA. A consultant in purchasing and supply-chain functions. Flying all over. Dad and I are so proud of what you've done, but more importantly, who you *are*. You are hardworking with a strong moral code. I just can't believe that you call us every week. You come to visit and bring us our favorite wine or help restain the picnic table. You are the one who remembers about Valentine's Day flowers. Dad and I often say, "We done good!"

Tee, we love you *thiiiiiiiiiiiiiiiiiiiiiis* much!

***

What do health-care experts write about sibling response to a chronically ill child in the family? Did the Hayles family experience what psychologists find in their research?

A chronically ill child can both unintentionally harm *and* help fellow siblings, according to Nancy Boyd Webb in *Helping Children and Adolescents with Chronic and Serious Medical Conditions.* In one study involving a child with diabetes, "it was found that siblings both *benefited* (with high levels of behavioral competence) and were *penalized* (by anxiety and low self-concept)."[7]

According to Webb, healthy siblings of a chronically ill family member often learn adaptability. They also realize that they are an integral, functioning part of the family process. According to a 2006 study by Roberta Woodgate of children with cancer, healthy siblings often understand that

---

7. Nancy Boyd Webb, ed., *Helping Children and Adolescents with Chronic and Serious Medical Conditions* (Hoboken: Wiley, 2009), 32.

the parent needs extra time with the sick child. However, the healthy sibling will at the same time feel left out and isolated.[8] Additionally, the healthy child can often feel sadness about his brother or sister's chronic illness. That sadness is often unrecognized by parents, which causes further stress in the healthy child. However, Webb indicates that "it would seem that children act to preserve families amidst a situation of being overwhelmed. . . . The healthy sibling does his or her part by laying [*sic*] low."[9]

When I think of Webb's words and my son Tee, I am again struck by how "textbook" Tee's growth into adulthood has been.

Around the time Tee turned sixteen, he had displayed a growing sense of responsibility in life. His grades rose to As and Bs. He became organized: his backpack was an orderly cataloguing of books; his bed was made; his assignments were completed on time. Tee began to garner attention that had inadvertently been pulled away from him. He became a superb swimmer, winning medal after medal. He excelled in the high hurdles in track—a sport that requires both speed and strength.

Tee's pattern in college continued. His grades moved to all As; he became president of his fraternity and vice president of the honors fraternity for business majors. He got runner-up for homecoming king, and all the while, a bevy of cute women flocked around him. I also remember Tee's college graduation vividly. He proudly wore the honors gold cord down the sleeve of his graduation gown. Four award medals hung around his neck. Tee was a star and in no one's shadow that day.

What would experts say about Tee's experiences being the big brother of a chronically ill child? Did he benefit, or was he penalized, as the textbooks indicate? Yes, and yes.

---

8. Webb, ed., *Helping Children and Adolescents*, 32.
9. Webb, ed., *Helping Children and Adolescents*, 32.

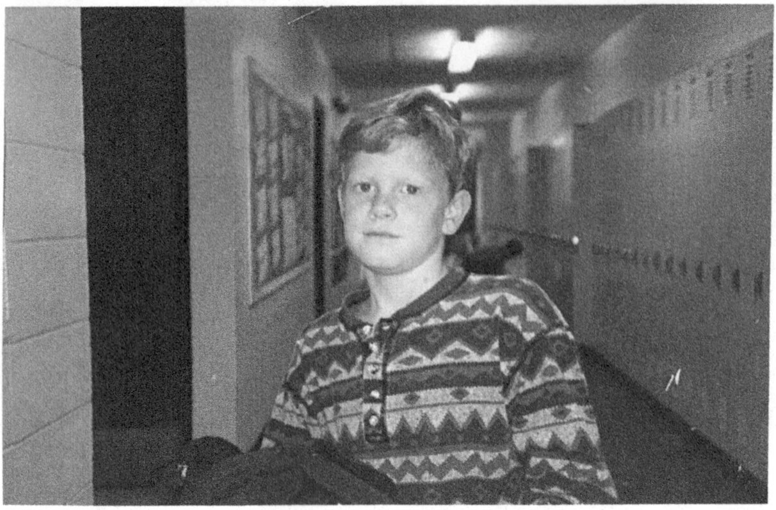

The shadow child

To this day, Tee pushes himself within the paradigms of success as defined by our family. Also, he is the epitome of the thoughtful, giving son. He never misses a birthday or a Christmas celebration. His gifts are considerate and unique. For instance, how many sons understand that a mother would love hand-blown wineglasses? On family vacations, Tee will go to market for fresh fish, making a fabulous dinner for the whole family. He'll call his grandma regularly. The list goes on and on.

Yes, growing up as a shadow child has given Tee some benefits. His accomplishments are what Western society often appreciates today. Quite often, individuals who are hardworking, educated, and people savvy are those who do well financially in the US. Additionally, as Tee worked to get out of Sammy's shadow, he discovered numerous personal skills—scholastic and athletic—that may have lain dormant otherwise. Tee also has a real appreciation for getting up each day in a life that is simply "normal." As a thirtysomething, he has been illness-free. He understands that many people—40 percent of the US population—are not so lucky; they have some type of illness, either temporary or chronic.[10]

The negative aspects of Tee's compensation are several. The young man acts according to what others want—not always what he wants. Additionally, he is still "in competition" with the world. Tee continually goes for a good-paying job, robust education, sporty cars, gorgeous women. Can you blame him? The shadow child is tired of the shadows and just wants a little sun coming his way.

10. "About Chronic Diseases," National Health Council, July 29, 2014, https://nationalhealthcouncil.org/wp-content/uploads/2019/12/AboutChronicDisease.pdf.

21

Twists and Turns

Life was busy—really busy.

Martin ping-ponged back and forth from Paris in a company position that was continually growing. He had moved into site services, which meant he was in big trouble if the soup in the corporate cafeteria was cold or if the company helicopter had a "hard landing." My days at United Telecom—which had morphed into Sprint—were also full and exciting. You remember that "captain of industry" fascination I had? Well, work had *me.* My job was high risk and high reward. I loved working with programmers, Ernst & Young auditing, Legal, and Human Resources. However, if I screwed up, it meant scores of angry shareholders vibrating the phone lines and adverse tax consequences for the company.

Sprint periodically would gobble up a smaller company in the telecommunications industry. When that would happen, my department would inherit the new benefit plans to run. Sometimes, depending on how a plan was constructed, we could assimilate it into one of our own. More often than not, however, the new plan could not be legally molded into an existing one due to the Employee Retirement Income Security Act (ERISA). So our department added benefit plans like pearls on a necklace.

Fortunately, the drama queen in my department transferred to Human Resources to a position that paid more. We were lucky. I hired Shu Zhang to come in and tackle the SEC reporting for our benefit plans. Shu, a product of Mao Tse Tung's China, had a work ethic like no other. She cranked out perfect numbers and schedules, fending off our auditors from the local Ernst & Young accounting firm single-handedly. I'm not sure she ate or slept. Meanwhile, the rest of us polished and perfected a below-market stock purchase plan that became entirely automated. Our group chugged along like an Amtrak train heading to St. Louis. Occasionally, I could sit back for a minute in the hubbub and enjoy our efforts that took care of fifty thousand employees. I loved talking with our shareholders—benefits plans were not just a corporate function, but real help to real people. On a daily basis, I would talk with thirty or forty Sprint retirees, helping them with the purchase prices of their various stock plans and outlining the tax consequences of that sale of stock. More often than not, the Sprint stock plus Social Security benefits were how retirees planned to support themselves. Although I had enjoyed teaching junior high students and cheerleading those helping verbs, this job—this role—made me feel complete.

The home front was a hubbub of a different nature. By this time, 1998, Sammy had graduated to kindergarten after two years in preschool. "I was 'helded' back," he'd explain to everyone. And indeed, he had been. Sammy's brain wasn't the culprit—it was his body. Despite cornstarch, Citrucel, Tolerex, allopurinol for gout prevention, and quarterly blood work and ultrasounds, Sammy lagged slightly in physical development. Somehow, he remained unfazed by all this. Playdates and birthday parties sprang into his life like popcorn hoppin' out of a skillet. Sammy's trips to the school nurse for cornstarch were just part of the class routine. Also, his Mic-key button seemed no big deal to classmates. "It's kinda cool," said one of Sammy's classmates to me during a field trip. "You could drink a bunch of red Kool-Aid through your Mic-key and you'd never have to brush your teeth. Hey, I wonder if you could shoot stomach goo out of your button?"

Tee seemed to like sixth grade all right. He'd bring a wad of homework home each night. Amy would help tackle the math; I was vice president of book reports and social studies after dinner. We'd work on pop-top rockets and balloon hovercrafts. We'd practice on spelling lists. The words seemed to whiz through Tee's brain with no impact.

Mrs. Mann, Tee's teacher, was on her game. One day at work, I got a call.

"Tommy is struggling with his reading. Unfortunately, he is testing below the fifth-grade level. I can see that in class he's having trouble keeping up because of this."

I felt dismay and guilt and irritation, all rolled into one big smack. I had been a teacher, for Pete's sake. How had I missed Tee's problem with reading? Was I focusing too much on my career that stroked my ego and fueled my brain? Had Sammy been getting all my focus? How on earth was I going to fit this new *problem* into a schedule that was packed with work and dinner and blood work and Tolerex and homework and laundry and book reports and . . .

Mrs. Mann gave me the name of a nearby reading specialty clinic. I scheduled a half day off work to take Tee in for a battery of seventeen reading tests. *Seventeen.*

The resulting report indicated that Tee had dysgraphia as well as other reading issues I simply couldn't pronounce.

I learned that dysgraphia was a neurological disorder that impaired writing ability and fine motor skills, impacting the spoken and written understanding of a subject. After I got my arms around Tee's reading diagnosis, I arranged for Amy to pick him up from school each day at twelve forty-five, drive him to Reading Solutions, and return him to class by two fifteen or so. Five days a week—back and forth. Seven months of retraining. Retesting. Then—success. Tee finished sixth grade in June, reading at the eighth-grade level. I was thrilled; this was my child who seldom made waves and hid in the shadows. He had been suffering academically, and I hadn't noticed. My attention was focused, as always, on Sammy's well-being and work.

All should have been good, but it wasn't.

I dragged myself out of bed each workday morning at five fifteen, slurping down two mugs of liquid ambition to shake off the morning coma. Often, when I'd get up at three o'clock to do Sam's cornstarch, I'd toss for an hour, ruminating about a new tax issue or a disgruntled shareholder. Five fifteen would come screaming at me just an hour later. Then, there were the evenings:

> 6:00 p.m.: race in the door, kick off shoes, and debrief with Amy.
> 6:05 p.m.: hug-and-catch-up time with Sam and Tee.
> 6:30 p.m.: strip off the suitcoat and cook dinner.
> 7:00 p.m.: dinner with the family.
> 7:20 p.m.: short TV time for the boys. Do up dishes and pull out frozen meat for the next night. Throw in one load of laundry. Check backpacks for forms to fill out and sign. Dump out gamey gym clothes. Wash and fill up cornstarch containers.
> 7:45 p.m.: homework time with the boys.
> 8:00 p.m.: shower time for Sammy; mix up Tolerex; story time; start the Kangaroo pump.

8:20 p.m.: Sammy in bed. Begin Tee's shower.
8:30 p.m.: Tee's story time and hugs.
9:00 p.m.: laundry in dryer.
9:15 p.m.: prepare boys' backpacks and snacks for the next day.
9:30 p.m.: answer work-related email.
10:00 p.m.: a sip of wine and a chat with Martin.
10:30 p.m.: bedtime.
3:00 a.m.: middle-of-the-night Kangaroo pump check.
5:15 a.m.: back at it.

One night, I stared at the whirring goo of Tolerex in the blender, shaking out a new IV bag in readiness for the smelly mess. I was so tired. So tired. I just wanted to find the nearest bed, pull up the covers, and hide. What was worse, I realized that I was getting to see Sammy only two hours on a workday, and Tee only three. Martin and I only got to chat about half an hour a night. It didn't feel right. Not right at all.

Had my mother gone through this angst with me when she went back to teaching? She was lucky; she had gotten home at four o'clock each day. And there had been only one of me. And I had been healthy. And my dad didn't travel; he was home by five o'clock each day. But Mom had had a good teaching career—first high school and then as department head of a small Presbyterian college in Emporia. Wasn't that what a woman did? A woman became well educated and then cruised through a succession of good careers. A woman could have a great husband, children, and a demanding job, right? Plus, make cherry pies? I thought of my favorite song when I was a kid. Blasting at full volume on our stereo in Emporia, Peggy Lee would belt out the words to "I'm a Woman."

If my mother and Peggy Lee could do all this, I was evidently lacking as a woman. Would I have to make a choice between career and motherhood?

I didn't *want* to make a choice. I loved both.

***

It was time for another necessary conversation. Martin had gotten home from Paris Friday night. It was a peaceful Saturday afternoon, poplar leaves curling and flipping across our back deck. Tee and Sam were next door at Scotty's home, playing. The atmosphere in our home had simmered with an undercurrent of constant tension for months. Martin's work, my work, the kids. And the GSD. The GSD. That constant, unwelcome party.

"I can't do this much longer, Martin." I made a feeble attempt to scoop up a pile of newspapers. The house was a wreck of toys, drink cups, and soccer balls.

For the first time in our marriage, Martin and I began to consider a single-income future. We looked at Martin's job level—considerably higher than mine. I was fortunate to be a manager at Sprint, but the harsh reality of the 1990s was that only *two* women directors existed at corporate headquarters and only one female vice president. It didn't look good for me. I felt like a kid in a candy store, with my nose pressed against the corporate glass ceiling that still kept women in place. It made sense to have Martin continue to work, because his earnings potential was simply better. I still love Martin for the fact that he never assumed that *I* should be the one to stay at home. However, we both knew finance, and the numbers didn't lie. I didn't want to quit work—I loved the exhilaration of problem-solving and helping shareholders. But I was tired—so tired. Also, was I being a mediocre mother?

That Saturday afternoon, Martin and I grabbed notepads and scratched out ideas. Costs for me to work outside the home: Amy, gasoline, dry cleaning, suits, costly made-to-order food, biweekly housecleaning help. Wear-and-tear on the car; wear-and-tear on the family. What could we ditch in our lives? Keep the old station wagon forever. Scrap vacations. Eat more hamburger. Embrace Pizza Hut and ditch Crowder's Steak House. I could be the house cleaner and the errand runner. We could do this. We *had* to do this. However, I felt pangs as Martin and I discussed the options. Was this the role I was meant to play in life? Would I turn into a bathrobe-wearing, soap-opera-watching slob as a stay-at-home mom? Would my mind melt into mush as I devoured Nora Roberts's heaving-bosom novels? This was a new paradigm for me, and not a comfortable one. I was also afraid of what other career women would say to me. More importantly, I was truly afraid of what *I* would say to me. *Hmm, Janet. Not living up to your mother's image? Living life in a mediocre fashion? Letting your brain rot?*

***

I've been gone from my work now for twenty years, and I still miss it. I loved working with company programmers and lawyers to improve the benefit plans. I loved digging into sheets of data and figuring out patterns and flows. I loved helping employees in our department grow, get training, and get promoted. I loved helping the little old lady shareholders with their stock questions as they were trying to figure out their retirement. I loved getting up in front of shareholder meetings to discuss the next stock offering. I loved chatting with Bill Esrey, the CEO, as I huffed and puffed on the stair-stepper at the company fitness center. I loved it. . . .

Oddly enough, within two weeks of quitting my corporate job, I found that being a stay-at-home mom also gave me definition and challenge. Had that 1970s "I am woman; hear me roar" just been bunk? Had I been sold a bill of goods by popular culture?

I think so. When a woman has a demanding career, a marriage, one "normal" kid, and one with chronic issues, she can't do it all. Something will give. Typically, what gives is time spent with the spouse or the children. What also gives is the woman's sanity. A career is important, but so are spouses and children and mental health. When I take my last breath, I won't dream about Sprint's benefit plans. I'll think of Martin, Tee, and Sammy—my three loves. I'll think of our bike rides in Shawnee Park, cappuccino at Borders Books, and swim meets with wise old Catfish Charley.

I had to choose between an "official" career and family, and I feel to this day that I chose wisely given our circumstances. What's more important—I was so fortunate to even be able to make the choice in the first place. That's a blessing that I do not take for granted. Ever. With the decision to leave work, life would move forward now in a calm manner, surely, wouldn't it?

PART 3

WALKING FORWARD

22

Movin' On

I did not turn into a bathrobe-wearing, soap-opera-watching slob. I threw myself into number-crunching for the PTA. I coordinated the summer swim team at Lake Quivira. I worked with the kids at church to create Christmas pageants, herding thirty angels and shepherds onstage. I scrubbed toilets at home and simmered Bolognese sauce. I made one hundred scones for Tee's history unit on Victorian England. Every day was different, and every day was tied to my family. It was amazing. My brain still got challenged, and I got to flex my organizational skills. Who started the myth that the stay-at-home mom wears a cute apron and sips martinis? She puts in sixteen-hour days, yet they are very *good* days.

Most importantly, I took a deep breath for the first time in five years and watched Tee at soccer practice. I cheered Sammy as he played T-ball. He seldom made it to first base, but no matter. I sipped a good Chardonnay with Martin at the end of a busy day. It was great. Absolutely great. For the first time in years, our family felt the vibration of anxiety quietly slow down. And the old blue station wagon? It just got older. Didn't matter.

***

In the 1960s, Bob Dylan used to wail, "The times, they are a changin'." They certainly were for the Hayles family.

I'd been a stay-at-home mom for about six months. I still choked on the term, bristling if I got an eyebrow raise from a snooty female attorney at a neighborhood party. Maybe I was a family coordinator/love provider/dog walker/toilet scrubber? No label seemed quite adequate.

Martin came home one night, looking drawn in the face. During dinner, we witnessed a rousing discussion between the boys: "Boston *is too* in Texas. Boston baked beans—like what the cowboys eat over a campfire? That's *got* to be in Texas." Then, we supervised showers and story time. I loved this part of the day, because I could read stories to the boys without the nagging sense that I needed to plow through twenty emails afterward. I could simply *listen* to their ideas. We had some doozie concepts come out, too, as I learned to take time with my children. One night, I walked by Tee's room to hear, "Why do you have a beard under your arms, Dad? And how does Mrs. Parker know every time I've passed a note in class? I did *not* draw her with a gigandous wart!" However, Sammy was truly the question man. One night, he blurted out during story time, "Wait! Do you think we could connect the dots to Tee's freckles and draw a picture? If God doesn't need to take a bath, do you think he takes showers instead? Do snakes have ears?"

These questions always left Martin and me slightly breathless.

That night, Martin and I sat down for our usual chat with

some Three Buck Chuck, I imagine. Taking a sip of the wine, Martin's eyes twitched slightly at the slap of tannin. He took another sip anyway. "Well, stuff is going on at work," Martin finally got out.

"Stuff?" I was instantly alarmed. "Stuff going on" was never good.

"The company is moving its headquarters to New Jersey, and the president wants me to find new headquarters there and run day-to-day administration. I'd be in charge of the phone operators, flight operations, security, the cafeteria—all the things that employees get angry over. It would be a promotion for me. I've prayed over this job offer, but I want to see how you feel. If you're not on board, we won't do it." Martin handed me a glossy brochure on the wonderful state of New Jersey.

New Jersey! Oh, dear God. I walked to our bookcase and pulled out our atlas. *New Jersey . . . New Jersey . . . It's somewhere on the East Coast. Here it is. What? That tiny state? Does it even have* roads? *Looks like it could drop off into the Atlantic. Hmmmm . . . it's really close to New York City. All that crime. Hypodermic needles on the streets. Oh, but the Metropolitan Museum of Art. Broadway. Central Park. Ellis Island . . .* My mind flipped between excitement and dread.

Folks from Kansas are fairly certain that nothing exists other than Kansas. Why would you want to move and leave miles of rolling wheat and the smell of cattle dung? Besides, we are pretty sure that once you get to the Kansas border, the world is flat and you just drop into an abyss. Heaven knows what is in *New Jersey.*

"Let's think on this, and I'll do some praying for guidance too," I replied to Martin. My world paradigm was cracking. Why would you ever leave Kansas?

Martin and I have always been firm believers in divine nudges. Our spirituality has led us in certain directions, and those directions have been good. So, after about a week of listening—just listening to a God that no longer smote me but had walked with me through the rough GSD journey—I knew it. I felt it. New Jersey would be okay.

"How are we going to tell the kids about this?" I looked at Martin, swirling my Three Buck Chuck. As usual, Martin was prepared. By this time, Sam had moved to first grade and Tee was in seventh. It would be a tough time to move the kids from Kansas to New Jersey.

Martin came up with the idea of reading our kids a story about change. The prior week in a staff meeting, one of the managers had mentioned a book called *Who Moved My Cheese? For Kids.* Apparently, since quite a few families would be impacted by the upcoming corporate move, this book was supposed to help break the news to kids. The book was a parable of sorts, about two mice, Sniff and Scurry, and two little people, Hem and Haw, who lived in a "maze" and looked for "cheese" to nourish themselves. The "cheese" represented *what* these characters wanted in life, and the "maze" was *where* they would hunt for what they wanted. However, only one of the mice handled the process successfully, with minimal stress. The victor wrote his "ah-ha" on the maze wall.

A week later, Martin brought home *Who Moved My Cheese? For Kids.* After dinner, he gathered us in the family room.

"No homework tonight!" he announced. "I've got a special story to read to you all." Martin proceeded with the drama of the cheese. He was a good reader: I could almost see Hem and Haw blundering through the maze. The boys were riveted; even our new pup, Georgie, sat nearby, watching the family and gumming her stuffed squirrel.

Martin finished the book, preparing to tell Tee and Sammy about our move. "Well, guys, here's what's going to—"

Sammy blurted out in the middle of Martin's last sentence of the grand performance. "So, are we moving?"

How did Sammy *know*?

23

"Joisey"

New Jersey turned out to be the coolest thing since sliced bread.

We found a house in the town of Pittstown on the western side of the state, although I hesitate to use "west" and "east" when referring to New Jersey. With one good sneeze, you can head out of the Newark airport onto I-78 and be halfway to Pennsylvania. At any rate, the western side of the state had lower property taxes. Coming from Kansas, we wallowed in sticker shock at the New Jersey housing prices and taxes.

Our neighborhood in Pittstown consisted of twenty-eight homes surrounded by sod farms and cattle. I snickered the first five years in New Jersey when I said the word "Pittstown." The town made my hometown of Emporia, Kansas, look like a burgeoning metropolis. Pittstown had a bank, a deli, a bed-and-breakfast, and an old barn bearing a faded sign that said, "You R Here. So, This Is Pittstown." I could head north five minutes to the big town of Clinton, housing about ten thousand residents.

Clinton absolutely radiated cuteness. I would come into town for errands, driving slowly over an old metal bridge straight from nostalgic Christmas cards. I'd cruise slowly past a red gristmill from the 1700s. A slow-moving river meandered on either side of the downtown, complete with lazy kayakers and circling geese. It was like Norman Rockwell had painted broad strokes of charm with uninhibited excitement. The two blocks of downtown displayed brick storefronts, cute shutters, and planters bursting full of ivy and pansies. In springtime, the town streets became a magic fairyland of white cherry blossoms. In the winter, you could stroll by the shops, admire the twinkling white Christmas lights, and sip hot chocolate. While the typical small Kansas town sported a fly-specked Dairy Queen and a hardware store reeking of fertilizer, downtown Clinton had gorgeous shops filled with leather goods, Brighton shoes, and gourmet pistachio ice cream.

We landed in Pittstown just a few days before Valentine's Day 2000. Martin and I had planned on relocating in the middle of the school year so Tee and Sammy would make friends by summer. The kids' school was called Union Township—incorporating kids from kindergarten to eighth grade. I loved the place. The school was a throwback to the 1960s—a red-brick single-story affair with playgrounds and soccer nets. The inside of the school smelled vaguely of chalk, beanie weenies, and dirty sneakers. Everyone knew everyone in the school, and the lucky teachers only had about twenty children per classroom.

On day one at the new school, Tee and Sammy walked two doors down from our home and caught the 8:15 a.m. bus along with the rest of the neighborhood gaggle. They hopped with excitement, because they had never ridden a school bus except for occasional field trips. The boys' backpacks were filled with notebooks, approved snacks, and Valentine cards for each classmate. Not bad. The first day of school for the kids, and bada-boom bada-bing. A Valentine's party.

I called Mrs. Mintel at the close of day one, trying to contain my helicopter-ness. Not surprisingly, Sammy appeared at ease at the new school. He would walk down the hall to Mrs. Mason's office twice a day for his cornstarch.

I had met with Mrs. Mason, the school nurse, just a few days prior to discuss Sammy's cornstarch schedule and to bring in boxes of Argo starch and spare syringes. I provided her an ER instruction list, contact list, and snack/cornstarch schedule list. Mrs. Mintel had the instructions, too, as did the PE teacher. Awareness and education were crucial for Sammy's safety at school.

Mrs. Mason hailed originally from "Longah Islant," where she loved to go "down sho-ahh" to Cape May and drink "caughwwwfee." She was an island of motherliness in the middle of the school day. Kids came to her for headaches, scraped knees, test anxiety, and, well, cornstarch.

Tee, our stoic son, was *not* well adjusted at Union Township, I found out months later. He was a new seventh grader in a sea of kids who had known each other for six years. He was the newbie—the outsider from Kansas, wherever *that state* was. And Tee, not wanting to trouble Mom and Dad, just dealt with the loneliness. The shadow child was, as usual, lying low, quiet. And I didn't notice. Again.

***

The best part of Clinton and Pittstown was that Dr. Charles Stanley was only an hour and a half away at the Children's Hospital of Philadelphia. Quite accidentally, back in Kansas City, I had run across an article about Dr. Stanley. He was considered a GSD expert, and boy, did we need an expert. Dr.

Marris in Kansas City was technically expert, but he never explained anything to me. It was a "getting blood from a turnip" scenario. Within ten minutes of reading about Dr. Stanley and the Philly children's hospital, I called long distance and had made an appointment for late February.

We had only just moved to Pittstown when Sammy and I made the big drive to Philadelphia. Neighbors had instructed me to take County Routes 513 and 527, cutting diagonally across rolling Jersey sod farms to I-95 South. "This is fine!" I said to Sammy. "We can do this!" Actually, I had never driven in a city larger than Kansas City. Six-year-old Sammy busily turned the dials of the radio, trying to find the Red Hot Chili Peppers. As we got fifteen miles outside of Philly, traffic on I-95 began to crawl, snakelike. The highway was a series of ruts, blacktop patches, and orange barrels.

Yes! There's Exit 22 to downtown Philly. With my blinker on, I slowly edged to the right. A line of cars blocked the lane I wanted, like a crawling wall. "Sammy! Give 'em your cutest smile!" I waved to the drivers to my right, batting my eyelashes. We needed to get over a lane and fast.

Nothing. I was invisible. My exit was 200 feet away. Then 150. Then 100. *Okay, here it goes,* I thought grimly. Determined, I put my blinker on again, grabbed the steering wheel, and did a "Jersey Slide." Somehow, traffic parted like the Red Sea, as the angry Kansas mom plowed across two lanes to Exit 22.

"Hey, lady! Learn to drive!" one cabby yelled at me, gesturing rudely from his car window. I *may* have said, "Sammy, my goodness, look over there at the vintage red Corvette." I then flipped the cabby off with enthusiasm. Oh, my mother would *not* have been proud.

The Children's Hospital of Philadelphia is both a mecca of hope and despair.

The facility is massive, with parking garages that wind up fourteen floors to a nosebleed level. Shiny bright hallways take you to this elevator, and then down this corridor, and across this walkway, and down this escalator, then over to this waiting room, and into this door. Large silver mobiles slowly twist from the ceiling of the main hospital hallway. Rows of red-framed children's artwork line the halls.

Amidst this exterior cheerfulness, Sam and I sat in Endocrinology and saw children with issues. All kinds. Some kids were in wheelchairs with feeding tubes. Some had no legs. Some sat by the bells and slides of the activity walls, not knowing what to do with the toys. Some just lay, inert, in their parent's arms.

Sam didn't say anything as we trekked to Endocrinology and the labs that day, but he took it all in, his blue eyes wide and a little watery. Outside of a string pack filled with cornstarch and syringes, you couldn't tell there was anything wrong with him. I think, for the first time, Sammy realized he was blessed, although I'd never really heard him complain much. Yes, GSD was bad; it could kill you. But he could walk. He could think. He could go to school.

"Mom, I think I'm kinda lucky." Sammy ratted through his string pack for some crackers. We sat on a crinkly vinyl couch in the Endocrinology waiting room, leafing through *Duck Dodgers in Outer Space* for a few minutes. And then: "Sammy Hayles? Mrs. Hayles?"

Dr. Stanley and his PA, Linda Steinman, were an aura of light in the hospital. We met for an hour, where Sammy was gently poked and prodded, weighed and charted. But most importantly, Dr. Stanley and Linda talked to Sammy like the bright young man that he was. He wasn't GSD Specimen Number 24, but the official class clown of the Union Township first grade. He was a drum player and a skateboarder. He was a kid of a thousand questions.

Sammy and I went from Dr. Stanley to the blood-work lab to ultrasound. "We want Sammy to have quarterly lab work as well as the quarterly ultrasound. We'll see you back here in three hours to evaluate our results." The crinkly blue-eyed endocrinologist smiled at us and shook Sammy's hand. "Young man, we'll see you in a bit, okay?"

The phlebotomist captured five vials of Sammy's blood. I was amazed; Sammy had had blood drawn so often he could just nonchalantly observe the draw, while I would hold his other hand and hum *Yankee Doodle*, looking across the room to keep calm. Blood draws always made me think back to my five-year-old days in Hutchinson, Kansas. Mom used to take me to the Payne Clinic on Sixth Street for my annual vaccinations. The name still makes me laugh. I'd scream bloody murder, my hindquarters tensed up like a board to avoid the polio vaccination.

After an extensive ultrasound of the liver, kidneys, gallbladder, and bladder, we headed for a forty-minute play session with a child psychologist. Sam would be followed quarterly by Mrs. Henderson.

It's so true that kids with chronic illnesses or disabilities are at risk for psychological stress, as are their siblings and parents. Sharon Dempsey in *Extreme Parenting* indicates that "play therapy is recognized as being beneficial in helping children to explore issues affecting them. . . . The fear of hospital procedures and the uncertainty of the future create anxieties that can be explored through play therapy. . . . Through play, the child can communicate unconscious and conscious experiences and emotions."[1] I had learned through articles from NORD that GSD could be associated with a reduced quality of life as well as elevated levels of distress in both the afflicted child and his parents. Fortunately, the Children's Hospital of Philadelphia was no stranger to children with unique and devastating conditions. While the Hayles family played together, ate together, and hugged together, we didn't know if we were

1. Dempsey, *Extreme Parenting*, 111.

managing the collective stress of illness appropriately. Perhaps the therapist could help.

So I sat outside the therapy room, twisting my shoelaces and flipping through *Parenting Today.* Sammy *seemed* to be doing okay with stress, as far as I could tell. Each day, he'd burst in the door from school with Tee, talking nonstop as I fixed the boys PB&J or popcorn.

"It's not fair! I was five feet away from Kyle when he got in trouble for making fart noises. The teacher gave me a time-out too. I was *there,* but not *involved.* And I did *not* call Mrs. Decker a lard ass. Oh, here's my multiplication test. I got an A. Here's my spelling test. I missed one."

"Sammy, what are these five red tickets here in your backpack? What do they mean?"

"I dunno. They're from my teacher. Oh, Mom, Dan invited us over to rollerblade after school. Can we go?"

"Sure . . . for just a bit. Both of you—grab your kneepads and helmets. Sam, what do you need to do when you get home from school, *first*?"

"Cornstarch?"

"You bet. And at what time?"

"Uhhhh. Four o'clock?"

"You've got it, Sam. And here . . . help me rinse out today's starch containers and refill two of them. That's it. Wipe them really dry and place them rim down on this clean towel. I know you'll only be three doors away, but what do you need to do, *always*?"

"Fill my string pack with my cornstarch containers and bottled water? And wear it?"

"You betcha. And your next starch time is seven o'clock. Hugs and kisses, guys. Tee, you and Sammy need to be back at four forty-five to start homework, okay? Both of you: set your watch timers."

I was a believer in hands-on training with Sammy as well

as daily repetition of his cornstarch schedule. I wanted Sammy to incorporate his health care into his very being. It would have to be second nature, because no GSD cure was in sight. Careful management was our only hope. I remembered only too well my own father. He had neglected his type 2 diabetes, suffering from poor vision, a heart attack, and two failed kidneys.

Both boys tromped out the door, ready to rollerblade up and down Dan's driveway, taking miniature leaps off a cool one-foot ramp. I made a quick call to Sammy's teacher to learn about the proliferation of red cards in the backpack. Apparently, my young Sammy was quite social, and the teacher's presence at the front of the classroom was merely a suggestion that he should listen. Mrs. Mintel mentioned paper airplanes and spitballs too.

Before our visit to the Philly children's hospital, I had been fairly confident that Sammy's play therapy, class-clown role, plentiful social invites, and good grades meant that all was good in the ole noggin. But all the tests and follow-up discussion about Sammy's physical challenges were rather overwhelming and disconcerting. I had seen Sammy look worried when Dr. Stanley discussed starting him on allopurinol. Apparently, kids with GSD were at risk for gout. We were also going to get an appointment with a nephrologist at Children's Hospital to monitor Sammy's kidneys. Kids with GSD were *also* at risk for kidney complications. In fact, the blood lab gave us a huge neon orange collection container for a specimen collection. Dr. Stanley patiently told Sammy that the urine collection would measure how much creatinine and protein were processed through his kidneys. Then, there was also the discussion with Dr. Stanley about the ultrasound today that had revealed four adenomas on Sammy's liver.

"They're benign little growths on the liver, Sammy. Now, yours are about half an inch long, so they're tiny. They are called inflammatory adenomas, but they usually don't hurt anything. We will monitor them every three months here at the hospital with an ultrasound. If you measure and take your cornstarch very carefully, the little growths should just stay like they are. With blood-sugar control, your adenomas can stay the same, shrink, or disappear. Don't worry, Sammy—we will take special care of you."

Sammy and I sat there, a neon urine collection bottle and pages of data in hand. We both blinked, a bit stunned. Little tumors in my Sam's liver? How likely were they to develop into cancer? I looked over at Sam, who had peeled off his stinky blue sneakers and was rummaging in his backpack for food. Did he have any clue that he faced a lifetime of uncertain health? It seemed like the bad news just kept rolling in. Would we ever feel safe? Would we ever stop getting bad news?

That night, Sammy asked a heart-stopping question in the middle of *Harry Potter and the Sorcerer's Stone.* "Why did God give me GSD?" Sammy looked clear into my soul and waited.

The question seemingly came out of nowhere. I was floored for seconds but then remembered the flood of scary information that had hit us earlier that day at the hospital. I had felt so sick in my heart at the news of the adenomas. Tough facts were tough facts. GSD was GSD.

I had read in one of my parenting books that I had to be honest with my kids, but not overly dramatic. Sammy was smart, really smart, but he depended on the family for his sense of safety and his reality.

"Well, um." My mind raced. *How do you communicate tough medical information and theology? Know your child,* my gut told me. *Feed your child,* my gut had told me years ago, before Sammy had been diagnosed with GSD. I resolved to rely on my inner mom sense.

"Well, um," I repeated, stalling a bit. "Remember how we talked about how GSD happens? Dad has a defective gene and so do I. When you were created, there was a one-in-four chance that you could get GSD. But Dad and I had never heard of the condition. We didn't know we were going to give you anything bad. We love you and Tee more than anything, you know."

I took a deep breath while my mind zigzagged. "So, I don't think God 'gave' you GSD. It just happened. I think maybe because of GSD you will always be sensitive to other people and their health issues. You've been to the Philly children's hospital and seen all the kids with IVs or who can't walk, right? But here's the good news, Sammy. You were given a great brain. Maybe you have been created to do something wonderful. Something that requires a real compassion for others and a good mind. Do you think that might be true?"

Sammy reflected a moment. "I guess so. But it doesn't seem fair."

"No, it's really not fair, for sure. But you know, Dad and Tee and I are here for you, always. Always and forever. That's one thing you can count on." I gave Sammy a mama-bear hug.

Later that night, I was awakened by a stage whisper. *"Mom!"*

It was Sammy, standing by my bed with his comforter and dee dee. "Can I sleep down here next to you?"

"Sure." I made a comfy pallet on the floor right next to my bed, where I could reach out and touch Sam's cheek. Sammy hunkered down, sighing and rolling over into a child's oblivion. Within minutes, I heard "Mom!" again. Tee wandered over to our bed, his Ninja Turtle blanket in hand. Tee curled up next to Sammy. I touched the reddish curls. Georgie padded in moments later, snuggling next to the boys. The Hayles family slept in peace.

24

Dear Mr. God, It's Me, Sammy

Dear Mr. God,

Hey, it's me again. Sammy.

Mom and I went to the Philadelphia children's hospital today. I got to play with this cool machine in the lobby. It looked like a giant yellow bowl on a stand. Mom gave me a quarter, and when I put it on the rim, it went round faster and faster and faster, down into the insides of the thing. I tried to get the quarter out, but Mom said get your hand out of there what do you think you're doing because you might get bad germs and stop that right now. Let's go young man and I'm not going to say it twice.

I liked the doctor a lot because he has blue eyes like mine, except he has these lines around his eyes, like smiles have been carved into his face.

You'll be glad to know I was a good kid most of the day, but Mom wasn't. She made a bad sign to a taxi driver on the way to the hospital. I don't know what it meant except she wasn't waving at him. She said, hey look, Sam, there's a red Corvette, but there wasn't any red Corvette.

I know you're busy with all those other sick kids. Well, and you have to make it rain and be in charge of Easter and everything. You are a busy guy, but when you have a minute, could you get rid of my adenomas? They're bumpy things in my liver, and I don't want them. The doctor told me not to be scared, but I kinda am.

Do you think my mom is right? That because I have GSD, I'll grow up helping other people? It sounds like a good idea. But if you just want to cure me, that would be okay too.

Your friend,

Sammy Hayles

PS: Christmas is in ten months, and could you put me down for some new Rollerblades? I promise to not get any more red tickets at school or call the teacher a lard ass.

PS again: My brother, Tee, would like new Rollerblades too. Can you work him in? Also, please send Mom a message that broccoli is bad for us.

25

The Big Step

We had been in Pittstown for about five years when the boys' social schedules exploded. Football practice for Tee. Pizza parties. The sixth-grade spring dance with *real live girls.* Sammy's drum lessons and rollerblading escapades.

"Karthik invited me over for a sleepover!" Sam exclaimed one April day as he and Tee burst through the back door from school. By this time, Sammy was a cocky thirteen-year-old.

I dried my hands on an old, checkered towel; I had been elbow-deep in making meat loaf. Leaning on the kitchen island, I placed raw carrots and hummus out for the boys as my stomach did a one-eighty. I had known this question would come up soon with Mr. Social.

"Well, let me talk to Dad tonight," I replied, stalling.

Karthik lived catty-corner from our house, just a hop and a skip out our back door, with his father, Lakshan; mother, Amrita; and little sister, Anupama. Lakshan was a veterinarian.

Karthik, at age eleven, was bright—the kind of son everyone wanted to have. And Anupama, a round-faced five-year-old, would wander into my kitchen when Karthik was over. She loved to stand by the pantry door and widen her dark eyes. "I like Oreos!" she'd inform me, tilting her head and waiting.

"I promise we'll be in bed by ten." I came out of my reverie when Sammy started in on his arguments for the sleepover. "And Karthik's family is really healthy! They're vegetarian."

"So, no hot dogs over there?" I countered.

Sammy took another breath and went at it. "And you don't want me to be socially awkward. *And*, everyone is doing sleepovers. Tee gets to. And Tee gets all the pizza he wants." The marketing man revved up.

The guilt began rolling in. Tee was healthy, and Sam was compromised. Tee *did* get all the pizza he wanted at parties. With Sammy, I'd have him take two bites, then switch to carrots or cheddar Goldfish. *Walk away from the pizza,* I'd coach. *Just say no.* I sounded like Nancy Reagan in the midst of an antidrug campaign.

The next day, I called Amrita and told her Sammy had been invited to a sleepover that weekend at her house. Incredibly, Amrita knew about the proposed social event. Usually, we moms were the last to know, always bewildered when six kids would suddenly pop over. Within ten minutes, I wandered down to the backyard and into Karthik's home. Amrita and I reviewed Sammy's cornstarch schedule and his GSD symptoms. I had her phone number, and she had mine. Amrita had been a nurse before having children, and then there was Lakshan's veterinary background. Sammy's first sleepover would be in a medically informed household.

The night of the big sleepover, I stood in the backyard and watched Sammy trot to Karthik's house, the string pack bouncing on his shoulders. Sammy had his cornstarch schedule, cornstarch, glucose tablets, bottled water, snacks, timer watch, and walkie-talkie. I had the other walkie-talkie: Hayles Communication Central was operative. Was I being obsessive? Yes, definitely. Sammy had never slept more than fifty feet from me.

"Remember, now." I had kissed Sammy on his curly head as we packed up. "Cornstarch next at 8:00 p.m.; 11:00 p.m. and 3:00 a.m. are your bigger doses so you can sleep longer; 7:00 a.m. is a regular one. See the containers marked 'nighttime'? What do you do after the nighttime doses?"

"Call you on the walkie-talkie." Sammy impatiently glanced out our sliding glass doors, itching to see Karthik. The Mother Stuff was getting boring.

"Yes, please. If I don't hear from you, I'll traipse across the backyard in my pj's and curlers and knock on the basement door. You'll be embarrassed to death."

"Okay, Mom." Sammy trotted to Karthik's as I heaved an uncertain breath. Would Sammy get busy with video games and forget his cornstarch? Would he go berserk over cheese pizza? My baby had just walked out of my little control zone. Yet, it was time for the first sleepover to happen; it had to happen. This night would represent Sammy's first baby step to middle school, high school—maybe even college. I dared to dream a bit.

"The sleepover was the time of my life!" Sam burst in the next morning fairly early. I had been pacing the kitchen with a cup of Folgers but nonchalantly peeled a banana when Sam flew in. "We played *Grand Theft Auto III* and watched *Shrek*. It was awesome." What was awesome was that Sammy had done his cornstarch on time and had called me after each dose. A fun, uneventful evening was perfect for any kid. It was critical for a GSD kid.

I got half a hug in before Sammy started begging.

"Next week can I go to Michael's house?" Michael was across the street and down two doors.

"I think we can arrange that, after I meet with his mom, Michelle."

"And Josh wants me to come over too."

"Well, let's do a few more sleepovers in this neighborhood, first," I countered. Josh lived five miles away. "You have to be careful on the sleepovers, right? I need to feel comfortable with this. And *you*—you must become an expert in GSD."

"I'll be so responsible, Mom." And so, the sleepovers continued, at our house and all around the neighborhood. Within months, they happened all around the school district.

***

Sammy was thirteen when he got the flu. He vomited once and felt warm to my touch. I began giving him glucose gel immediately, but it flew back up within five minutes. After the second vomit, I grabbed Sammy's string pack and began loading up supplies: our ER instruction letter from Dr. Stanley, cornstarch, water, syringes, glucose gel, and healthy snacks. We roared fifteen minutes over to the Readington Medical Center, the nearest hospital.

I had always liked the hospital. It was new and friendly, with polished floors and pink-smocked volunteers. However, it was not a place where you'd go for heart surgery or GSD.

Sammy and I screeched into ER about seven o'clock that evening. Martin stayed home with Tee, heating up beanie weenies and supervising homework. I imagine that our new pup curled up on the kitchen floor nearby, aware that life was not right.

The triage nurse checked me in. Slowly. So very slowly.

I gave her insurance information. I showed her the ER letter. I filled out symptom information. I dug my nails into my palms. The nurse painstakingly took Sammy's temperature, blood pressure, weight, blood-oxygen level, and glucose. The minutes crawled as Sammy's eyes began to glass over and his head drooped.

"His glucose is at seventy-two," the nurse announced to me with a bit of contempt, as if to say, *Lady, this place is for emergencies.*

"Yes—I know. I've been giving Sammy glucose packets for the last hour. But when he has the flu, his lactic acid will rise, and the rest of the blood profile will start to collapse. See here? On this letter from Dr. Stanley at the Children's Hospital of Philadelphia. The Children's Hospital . . . agghhhh!" *Don't get witchy with this woman,* I thought. *Calm yourself. Calm yourself.* "Sammy has glycogen storage disease. We need to act fast—he could go into shock." I tapped the ER letter for emphasis and wiped my watery eyes. I was not going to panic.

The nurse seemed unimpressed as she called for a gurney for Sammy. Clearly, I was not a doctor and was therefore uninformed. Clearly, Sammy was only thirteen and therefore uninformed. Clearly, Sammy was not bleeding from stab wounds and was therefore not an emergency. However, I could see my son sinking into shock, his eyes dull and hollow. *I knew my son, and I knew GSD.*

Two minutes. Four minutes. How long could it take to get a gurney? Was I in an emergency room or in a darn parking lot? I looked around the ER waiting room. Two other patients were restlessly flipping through *Golf Digest* and *House Beautiful.* A fly buzzed frantically against one of the windows.

It took a full hour and a half before Sammy and I were admitted into the bowels of the ER and into a treatment room. Just in time, a nurse started an IV bolus of glucose and Anzemet into the crook of Sammy's right arm. Sammy's face had become pasty white—his eyes closed and skin clammy. Before we finally got an IV delivered to the room, I had been trotting up and down the hall, waving my emergency forms in general panic. I flagged down every nurse, doctor, and custodian I could find. "Someone's coming in to help soon," they all soothed me. After the bolus of glucose began to provide life-giving fluid to Sam, a nurse then set the Kangaroo pump clicking and whirring. Within thirty seconds of the bolus, Sam perked up, like a computer rebooting. Two blue eyes fluttered at me and opened in confusion. I rubbed my teen's forearm gently and gave him tiny sips of water and cheddar Goldfish. "Let's try a little cornstarch in thirty minutes and see if you can hold it down." My baby.

"Sammy, we are so lucky that you got the IV in time, because it saved your life. If you're off in college and this happens again in an ER room, grab your ER form and pretend to have a seizure if you get ignored. I might not always be with you, and even medical staff don't always realize how quickly things get dangerous for someone with GSD. When you get to a certain level in your blood sugar, you simply can't do anything for yourself."

"I got it, Mom. I got it." Of course, Sammy did.

26

More Steps

I always say, if you want an interesting life—raise a couple of boys.

I had been trying for months to get Sammy organized for school, but to no avail. Each Friday afternoon when Sammy would burst into the house, I could see that his backpack was expanding like a container of Jiffy Pop. A sour, musky smell would waft out. Against my better judgment, I'd dump the contents, discovering a ten-day-old container of banana yogurt, vibrant with moldy blues and greens. I'd pull out tightly wadded-up gym clothes, red plaid boxers, and one aqua sock with lace on it. Boxers? Whose boxers? And, more importantly, whose sock? Then, I'd hit the motherload. There would be a pile of mushy notes in the bottom of the pack—from teachers, the PTA, and assorted girls. Note One: "Mrs. Hayles, you have missed a vital PTA meeting regarding gift-wrap sales." Note Two: "You have missed a vital PTA meeting regarding the content of hot dogs in the school cafeteria." Note Three, from Mrs. Harding, your son's seventh-grade teacher: "Please note: Sammy has received four red tickets this week." Note Four: Mrs. Harding regrets to inform you that "Sammy is not working up to his potential and is extremely social." That's news? Note Five: Lorie writes, "I heart you!" Note Six: Stacey writes, "I heart you!" Okay, Lorie and Stacey, back off. Go "heart" some other kid. This is my son you're talking about. I decide that ignorance is indeed bliss, dunking the morass of notes into the trash.

Next, the grumbling would begin. One morning, I visited with Sam as he ate his scrambled eggs. Between mouthfuls, I heard. Boy, did I hear it.

"I don't know *how* the school expects us to get up so early and function properly. Don't they understand that we teens have special circadian rhythms? We need to start school at ten o'clock! And *how* am I supposed to survive on a slice of pizza, limp broccoli, and canned cling peaches? I need some decent brown rice to properly bulk up for my weight training. And this homework load! What's up with this busy work? Quadratic equations? *When* am I going to use that in my *real* life?"

Sammy would rev up like a preacher at a Wednesday night tent revival.

"And you know what? My science teacher actually took off seven points on Friday's test because of *spelling errors*. Spelling isn't supposed to count in science class! And did you know that we have to build a bridge that weighs only one hundred grams? But it has to support one hundred pounds. This is ridiculous!" My son finally took a breath.

"When is the bridge due?" I calmly asked the drama queen.

"Thursday," he whined between gulps of cornstarch.

Oh, great. Today was Tuesday. So it began.

***

Sammy was best buds with Josh at Union Township. Josh was a bit burly, athletic, and smart to boot.

Sammy burst in one day from school with his usual fan of red tickets from the teacher, notes from girls, complaints, stories, and requests. "Hey, Mom," he managed to get out between bites of his snack. "Josh asked me to go to a thing with him Sunday afternoon at his church."

Evidently "a thing" was something good because Sammy seemed so excited. Sunday came, and I busily packed up Sammy's pile of supplies into his string pack.

As Sammy later told me, for that special Youth Day, the church youth group leaders had rented a bouncy house and set up an obstacle course. A cotton-candy machine spit out pink fluffy magic in the church side yard, and popcorn scented the air. Over in another corner, church dads grilled hot dogs for the kids, and moms set out potato salad, baked beans, and cupcakes with a blue frosting cross on each.

After a frenzy of bouncy-house jumping and hot dogs, thirty sweaty kids tromped into the church. A young man stood at the altar, his curly brown hair just grazing his collared white shirt. His eyes were heavy lashed, earnest. He looked like a twenty-first-century Jesus, if Jesus had insisted on shopping at Polo.

"Boys and girls," he began, spreading his palms out to the gathering. "I know you think church is just for old guys and that Jesus is for losers. But do you want to be a winner? *Do you want to be a winner for Jesus?*" The young man brushed back his wavy brown hair and narrated his story. He had been with a biking crowd, spending his days drinking and drugging. Until one day, he had rested on a rock near a wheat field by Wellington, Kansas. There, he had seen Jesus in the field and had changed his life.

Electricity and spirituality sizzled through the air. "Yeah, yeah!" the kids echoed back. Sammy settled his sweaty back into the pew, filled a cornstarch container with water, gulped the chalkiness down, and drifted into a daydream. . . .

Later, at home, Sam told me that during the revival, he had begun thinking about his life's project: building a hovercraft. This invention had been an obsession for months. Sammy and I would wander through Home Depot for two hours at a time, while the young inventor selected this bolt and that cabling and those sheets of tin. Using our leaf blower as a propulsion device, Sammy was positive he could build a hovercraft and sail over to Karthik's house, magic-carpet-like. He could take our new pup's droppings and zoom over to the science teacher's yard, scattering them like confetti. The possibilities were endless and exciting. . . .

"You all stand up!" the young Jesus-man beckoned. "I say, stand and come on down!"

Sammy jolted back into reality, his daydream disappearing into the mist of his brain. As he told me, all he had heard was "Stand up," so Sammy rose uncertainly. He felt something was amiss when he heard people begin to clap all around him. Looking around, he realized that no one else was standing. No one. Out of two hundred people.

"Let's hear it for this young man, here. Come on down! Son, can you tell all these fine folks here that you've given your heart to Jesus? Everyone, let's hear a big *Amen*!"

Sammy blinked, ending up stunned and alone at the front of the church as the congregation applauded. The next thing he knew, he was signed up with a church sponsor. Fifteen church members came to the front of the church to lay their hands on him, praying for his sins, especially for all his red tickets from his teacher. In the midst of a big daydream, Sammy had been saved.

***

As best as I could tell, Sammy's church experience bounced off him like a tennis ball. The church members had loved him, Sammy told me that night. However, he never went back to the church, despite frequent offerings of picnics, softball teams, and youth camps. Instead, Sammy seemed to take on spirituality as I had as a kid. He, too, just wanted to get through life without being "smote" by God. I guess he felt GSD had smacked him enough.

***

It was about a week later that our family got an exciting pamphlet in the mail. Emblazoned across the front, it said, "Enroll *now* for the Institute for the Gifted summer camp!" Ooooh. Summer classes at Bryn Mawr, Pennsylvania. Ivy-covered stone walls. Classrooms reeking of academia. Hands-on science. I wanted to go to camp too.

That evening, I slid the glossy pamphlet over to Sammy at the dinner table. Tee was going to work that summer at ShopRite in the produce department, to help pay for Eleanor, his four-wheeled pride and joy. The vehicle was silver and had red calipers—the coolest of cool. Sammy was too young to work, of course, but I had a household rule: no more than two hours per day of video games. Each boy had to work, play outside, or take classes.

"See, Sammy? You'll share a dorm room with a friend. You'll have classes and recreational time each day, plus art projects, improvisation, and campfires. . . ."

Sammy interrupted my spiel, meatballs skewered on his fork. I absentmindedly took my own fork and gently poked his elbows off the table. Fancy-pants camp or no, manners were manners in our house.

"I wonder if I can build my hovercraft there," mused Sammy. "Hey, I wonder if *girls* will be there?"

"The brochure says coed," I replied. That cinched the deal. Girls and three weeks without parents. The possibility of hovercraft invention. It would be glorious.

The next day, it hit me. What had I just committed to? Sure, Sammy had done about twenty successful sleepovers by this time, but Bryn Mawr was another deal. The campus was almost two hours away. A lot could happen in two hours. Also, it was three weeks long: *five hundred and four hours* during which Sammy would have to remember cornstarch, alarms, class schedules, and diet restrictions. It was a lot for a thirteen-year-old.

I took a deep breath and called the toll-free camp number the next day.

"Ah. Will there be a nurse on campus? She's one building over from the dorms? Can I get her name and office number? What about getting a few special food items during the meals? You have gluten-free? Oh, that's great. What about sugar-free alternatives? Wonderful. Okay, here's my charge card number. . . ."

My next call was to Mrs. Meeks, the summer camp nurse at Bryn Mawr. Her friendly voice reminded me of Mrs. Mason, the loving school nurse at Union Township.

"Yes, Mrs. Hayles, we do have some children at summer camp with medical needs. Let's see. I think in the June session we have twenty-five children total. Two use an EpiPen. Bee and food allergies. I've got one with exercise-induced asthma, and one with type 1 diabetes. No, I've never worked with a child with GSD, but tell me about it."

Mrs. Meeks listened intently on the other end of the line. I went through the basics of Sammy's condition and care routine. Did she think she could work with us to help Sammy go to camp? Could Martin and I drive to Bryn Mawr before camp to go over information with her and form a game plan for nighttime cornstarch?

While we traveled to Bryn Mawr, Tee was to spend two days with his friend Brett. Brett's dad had dirt bikes, and the three would head out to zoom trails each day. Brett's mom was an apple pie–baking, hug-on-you-in-her-floured-apron kind of mom. On the Big Planning Day, Martin, Sammy, and I hopped in the car to meet with Mrs. Meeks. I was all a-flutter with excitement for Sammy, yet filled with fear too. I loved control, yet we were moving away from control—again—because we had to for Sammy's growth.

Bryn Mawr and Mrs. Meeks did not disappoint. Martin, Sammy, and I walked across a grassy campus and through a dignified granite archway of rocks into the nurse's office. After an hour of reviewing Sammy's forms, showing off his Mic-key button, and hearing a vigorous discourse on how to build a hovercraft, it was set. The Plan. Mrs. Meeks took her place alongside the other angels I had met thus far in life: Retha, Dr. Stanley, Amy, and Mrs. Mason.

As we discussed with Mrs. Meeks, Sammy would set his alarms at nighttime for larger cornstarch doses that would buy him four hours of sleep at a time. After each nighttime dose, Sammy would call the nurse on her dorm-room phone, using his new cell phone. If she did not get a call, she would physically head to Sammy's room to make sure the dosage had happened. This nighttime routine meant that Mrs. Meeks would set her alarm, too, every night, for three weeks.

I pulled on a cuticle nervously. "Maybe we should call Sammy, too, each night? Just to make sure?" I poked Martin to make my point.

"Mom, we've got it. Sammy is responsible, and I'm responsible. I'll call you the first morning of camp to let you know how it's going." Mrs. Meeks looked at me with sympathetic eyes; she was a mom too.

We lined up the supplies on Mrs. Meeks's office shelving. Twenty-five boxes of cornstarch, sugar-free Citrucel, plastic spoons, syringes, tubing, bottles of water, extra plastic containers, Level Life glucose gel, Goldfish crackers, allopurinol, oral Zofran for nausea, and an extra Mic-key button. Phone contact list, ER instruction list, cornstarch schedule. Extra timers. That was it. Mrs. Meeks's shelving was ready for end-times.

A week later, Martin, Sammy, and I made the trip back to Bryn Mawr. As we got "the baby" settled into his room, I compulsively laid out spiral notebooks, pencils, and cornstarch supplies. I placed two weeks' worth of shorts, tops, and underwear in his drawers. I hung up towels in the bathroom and generally obsessed. Toothbrush: check. Comb: check. Antibacterial hand wipes: check. Had we forgotten anything?

"Janet, calm down." Martin looked at me, shaking his head. He was always patient and philosophical. "We're leaving Sammy at Bryn Mawr with a nurse three hundred feet away. He's not in Outer Mongolia." Martin was right, of course. In two weekends, we would head back to Bryn Mawr for Parents' Day. I could swap out fresh clothing then, eat s'mores at the campfire, and watch the kids do their improvisations. This was not Outer Mongolia. But still—my baby would be almost two hours away from me. It was a scary first.

I gave Sammy one last hug before he and his new roommate, Kim Lee, dashed out the door to the first organized event of the camp: Frisbee tag, followed by a picnic dinner, a campfire, and a storyteller from nearby Haverford.

"Remember to—" I started to remind Sammy of his next cornstarch time.

Martin touched my arm. "*Stop,* Janet. Sammy set his watch alarm with me while you were hanging up towels in the bathroom. He's playing Frisbee right out there. See? Two hundred feet from his cornstarch supplies. His room key is on a lanyard around his neck. There are three teachers out there. Let it go."

The control freak in me softened a bit. I took one last desperate look around the dorm room, smoothed Sammy's bedspread compulsively, and headed off campus, grabbing Martin's arm for support. The drive home was long and endless, as mile after mile separated us from our child. Our child with a chronic illness. Our child who couldn't survive one night of missed cornstarch. Was this next step to independence okay?

***

That night back in Pittstown was also long and endless. I finally slept at about midnight, waking up automatically at 3:00 a.m. I had gotten up at that time for years, and twenty years later, I still wake up at 3:00 a.m. in hyperalert mode. That night, I eased out of bed, wandering down the hall to Sammy's room. His Rollerblades leaned in one corner. I opened the top drawer of Sammy's dresser. Pogs and Beanie Babies. The faded blue dee dee, long forgotten. I looked over to Sammy's bathroom, his toothbrush holder empty, crumpled red boxers on the floor. Was Sammy up right now, doing his cornstarch? The sixty miles to Bryn Mawr seemed so far, so far.

***

> Dear Mom,
>
> You never told me being a mom was so hard!
>
> I wrote you last week about Sammy's first time to go to camp. It's a lovely place, and thank goodness, there's a fantastic nurse there! She called me the first morning of camp. Somehow, I think she knew I was pacing the night before at 3:00 a.m. Well, I *was* up, looking at Sammy's dee dee and sniffing a bit. Mom, he's growing up to be such a bright,

funny, ornery kid. Can you believe he's as tall as I am?

The cornstarch routine at Bryn Mawr is going fine, according to Mrs. Meeks. Oh—she's the nurse. Can you believe she sets her alarm each night to make sure that Sammy has done his cornstarch? I'm going to write the director of the summer program and tell her what a dedicated person Mrs. Meeks is.

For Parents' Day, we got to come up for a picnic and look at the art projects. I'll never tell Sammy this, but when it comes to art, he'd better not make it his day job. I looked at his watercolor painting, hanging neatly with the rest of the kids' artwork. I know you can't say, "What is this supposed to be?" But really, Mom, what *was it supposed to be*? Sammy had painted a big red circle on a black background. That's it. A red circle. The title written on the painting was *My Cornstarch*. Hmmmm. Makes me think. Makes me worry. I'll talk to the therapist at CHOP about this. I have to say that, on a brighter note, Sammy's improvisational skills were amazing. He's so quick. Sammy's skit group did a scenario where two of them were in a taxi, and he was the driver from "Joisey" with plenty of attitude.

At the end of the three-week camp, Martin, Tee, and I hauled Sammy home. The back of the station wagon was filled with stinky laundry, art projects, and several notes from *girls*. The front of the station wagon was filled with victory. Sammy had successfully managed his health care for three weeks. In the meantime, Tee had reigned king at home. We had cooked lasagna and tacos for big brother. We had rented his favorite movies, including a remake of *Teenage Mutant Ninja Turtles*. He was taking a week off work and about to go to soccer camp. The Hayles family felt almost "normal."

27

Our Saint with the Knee-High Cast

Dr. Stanley looked at Sammy with his kindly blue eyes. "Would you consider doing this?"

I looked over at Sammy, who at age thirteen in 2005 was so tall that I looked eye to eye at him. This was the kid who supposedly would have subnormal growth. Sammy gazed at Dr. Stanley with an expression of interest. The three of us were standing in an exam room at the Children's Hospital of Philadelphia after an ultrasound, bone scan, blood work, and McDonald's.

"We really need smart young people like you to help with research on GSD," continued Dr. Stanley. "Wouldn't it be great to help with a new type of cornstarch? One that would allow teens like you to sleep seven hours at night instead of only four? Plus, you would really get to know Dr. Weinstein and his staff. I consider Dr. Weinstein the top expert in the world on GSD. That's all he does. He lives it and breathes it."

Dr. Stanley had just told us the devastating news that he was retiring from endocrinology at the age of seventy. The new endocrinology department head had little experience in GSD. Unfortunately, the Hayles family would have no expert close by to turn to.

I looked again at Sammy, who, in a single, fluid movement, poured water into a cornstarch container, shook it vigorously, and gulped it down. It was 3:00 p.m., and Sammy's watch had beeped. Sammy nodded to me, *Yes, I'll do the study,* swiping a cornstarch mustache off his lip. He pawed in his backpack for saltines.

"Let me talk to Sammy on the drive home." I rose, shaking Dr. Stanley's hand for the last time. "I am so grateful to you. Sammy is doing so well. He's doing sleepovers and did a camp at Bryn Mawr. Before long, he'll be learning to drive. Then maybe college. We're on a good road to independence."

Dr. Stanley stood and shook my hand. Sammy looked down, embarrassed, hesitated a second, and dove in to give Dr. Stanley a big hug. The doctor beamed. I swear I saw just a hint of a tear in one eye. "Sammy, I'm going to read about you one day in some professional journal. Keep studying, young man."

That night, the family gathered over dinner as we all shared our day. Mostly, we took turns sorting through the materials Dr. Stanley had given us that afternoon. It was exciting stuff. Really exciting.

We learned that Dr. Weinstein was a pediatric endocrinologist who had specialized in GSD the past twenty years. We had never heard of him! As a fellow at Harvard University, Weinstein became intrigued by GSD—"this disease that no one else was touching."[1] Weinstein moved to Florida in 2005 to work with the Gene Therapy Institute to develop genetic

---

1. Margaret A. Chen and David A. Weinstein, "Glycogen Storage Diseases: Diagnosis, Treatment and Outcome," *Translational Science of Rare Diseases* 1, no. 1 (August 2016): 45–72.

therapies for GSD. I scanned through the information further. "At present, he and his small staff operate on part of a floor at the University of Florida hospital in Gainesville. Dr. Weinstein sees approximately five hundred patients each year, including those from forty-nine states and forty-five other countries."[2] I read these words to the family, as a bit of hope flamed in my heart. "Oh, guys, listen to this." I read further. "'Iris Ferrecchia is a nurse for Dr. Weinstein. She has four grown children, three of whom have GSD.'[3] Oh, my. Here's what Iris says. 'When you have a doctor who cares so much, it's easier to have kids with it [GSD] because you don't feel like you are alone. . . .'"[4] Apparently, one of her sons needed a liver resection because of tumors. "Listen to what Ferrecchia says!" I waved another page of information at the family. "'I felt like I needed a doctor at 2:00 a.m., and [Weinstein] answered the phone.'[5] The nurse adds in her comments that Weinstein is often at the office until midnight; he is known to sleep just a few hours a night. . . . Dr. Weinstein is an interesting combination of science and love."[6]

"Yeah, Mom. Let's do this." Sammy shoveled in mashed potatoes with enthusiasm. "*I* can be a science experiment." Testing a new type of cornstarch wasn't exactly like building a hovercraft, but still, I could tell Sam was intrigued.

"And Sam. Are you okay with what it says here in the information? You'll be in the GSD wing of the University of Florida's hospital while I'll be across the street at the Holiday Inn at night. Three days, it says here. A get-acquainted meeting with Dr. Weinstein and staff first. That night, after dinner, a nurse will insert a port into your arm. You'll drink a dose of

---

2. Chen and Weinstein, "Glycogen Storage Diseases," 45–72.
3. Kristine Crane, "UF Pediatrician Earns Global Recognition for Treating Rare Disease," *Gainesville Sun*, January 9, 2013, https://www.gainesville.com/story/news/2013/01/09/uf-pediatrician-earns-global-recognition-for-treating-rare-disease/31841484007/.
4. Crane, "UF Pediatrician Earns Global Recognition."
5. Crane, "UF Pediatrician Earns Global Recognition."
6. Chen and Weinstein, "Glycogen Storage Diseases," 45–72.

regular cornstarch, but at eleven o'clock, you'll drink the experimental stuff. It says here . . . oh, where is it . . . the new starch is a high amylopectin—a high molecular weight. You can keep your port in during the day because they'll tape your arm up really well. Then, we can take a taxi to nearby museums or something. We just have to be back at the hospital by seven o'clock. Yes, that means TGI Friday's chicken fingers, young man! You'll go through the same routine the second night. The third morning is a debriefing on your medical data."

"Why do I have to get a port in my arm?" Sam didn't seem afraid, just irritated.

I flipped through two more pages of information. "It says here that all through the night, monitoring equipment will track your blood sugar and lactic acid minute by minute. Whenever your blood sugar drops below seventy, the testing ends. You'll take a dose of your regular cornstarch at that time, but the IV monitoring will continue until after breakfast that morning. You'll have a continuous record running. So, are you okay with all of this?"

"Yeah, this will be cool."

Cool, indeed. Sammy could help with GSD research, becoming the first "guinea pig" in history to test the new type of cornstarch. Even better—Sammy could become a patient of the top GSD expert in the world.

***

The University of Florida and Dr. Weinstein's GSD research floor were amazing. How could a huge hospital and rows of research labs feel so welcoming? It was Dr. Weinstein and his staff. They were simply wondrous.

Sammy and I flew into Gainesville midafternoon for our three-day beta testing. At the hospital, we wound our way through hallways and elevators until we got to the GSD stomping grounds. I glanced to the right and left as we headed to Sammy's room. Hmmmm. A GSD baby and her parents. A teenager. A twentysomething? Patients of all ages were waiting for GSD hope.

I remember that a freckle-faced nurse wheeled in a small cart with GSD-approved snacks and drinks. Sammy consumed cheddar Goldfish with great relish, busily checking off selections for dinner. Check. Check. Check. Check. Being a GSD test subject was hungry business, indeed. Or, maybe it was nerves. Or, maybe it was just being almost fourteen.

Dr. Weinstein breezed into Sam's room about five o'clock, dressed in a white button-down shirt and a loosened tie picturing Tweety Bird. He clomped over to a chair near Sam's bed. Wow. A bright blue cast went from his toes to his knee on the right leg. Dr. Weinstein extended his hand.

"Mr. Sammy. I'm so glad you were able to come and help with our GSD beta testing. Can I sit and visit for a while?"

"Uh, sure. What did ya do to your leg?" Sammy was not one to beat around the bush.

"Well, I've got a patient from Clifton, New Jersey, and his insurance company is refusing to pay for his GSD blood work and treatments. I lost my temper last week and kicked the wall of my office. I've been trying to help the family get medical coverage, and nothing is working."

Wow. Dr. Weinstein was a man of passion and caring.

I sat across from Dr. Weinstein with my yellow legal pad, busily writing down the conversation with Sam. In an hour, the two talked of Sam's career interests. Who knew Sam wanted to be a lawyer some day? I mean, Martin had gone to law school, but Sam? Who knew the kid wanted to perform improv? Who knew he liked Samantha? Furthermore, who *was* Samantha? Then, Dr. Weinstein drew out a diagram of how Sam's liver processed—or mostly *didn't* process—glycogen into glucose. The two talked of high school and college and the inherent risk of alcohol. Apparently, Sam could face a double whammy: alcohol would inflame his already-challenged liver. Too much alcohol could also make him miss his cornstarch alarm. And with weight training—steroids were especially lethal to folks with GSD. Unfortunately, I learned that some weight-training supplements contained small bits of steroids and had to be avoided at all costs. I scribbled away, amazed at the vast amount of information that flowed from Dr. Weinstein. Where had this saint been all my life? I glanced at Sam. He was engaged with the earnest doctor as information simply flowed.

With the excitement of a twelve-year-old, Dr. Weinstein thumped into Sam's room the morning of day two, sporting a Tasmanian devil tie this time. He had a koala bear wrapped around his stethoscope, to boot.

"Great news!" he announced to the two of us. "Guess how long you went last night on the *new* starch?" Dr. Weinstein didn't wait for an answer. Waving sheets of data, he exclaimed, "Eight hours! You went eight hours! That's groundbreaking. Now, we'll need to see how you do tonight. And, of course, the new starch will be tested on scores of GSD patients of all ages. We'll do refined dosing tests in a few months. I hope you'll come back to help us, because we sure can use young people like you."

Mid scrambled eggs, Sammy was full of smiles. He had *never* had eight hours of uninterrupted sleep.

At the end of the three days at the University of Florida, Sammy also received a two-week nutrition plan for GSD, as well as a detailed cornstarch dosing schedule based on his age, weight, and activity level. Cornstarch had to be measured precisely for each dosage, something that I hadn't been doing so carefully. I hadn't realized that too much cornstarch could elevate Sammy's blood sugar, but too little would allow the sugar level to drop. On day two of the GSD study, Sam's port arm was securely wrapped; he pulled on a long-sleeved checkered shirt. Apparently, it was one *Samantha* liked. We headed two floors down to the hospital pharmacy to buy a glucometer and test strips for blood-sugar testing. Then, according to Dr. Weinstein's instructions, we walked three blocks west of the hospital to a local head shop. There, amidst the marijuana pipes and bubblers, we bought a really good gram scale. A proper gram scale has a "tare" function, so that the weight of the plastic container does not factor into the weight of the cornstarch. The dosage for Sammy would be precise—thirty-six grams per dose during the day; sixty-five at night.

In thinking about those three groundbreaking days in Gainesville, I remember the practicality of Dr. Weinstein's help. We received custom-tailored ER instructions on his letterhead, a revised dosing schedule, and a travel letter for the TSA ("Uh, young man, what are those little containers of white powder in your backpack?"). We had pages of nutritional information and easy-to-understand GSD medical data. One of the nurses gave us an application to join Medic Alert so that Sammy would have a life-saving data card in his wallet at all times. As it turns out, Medic Alert could even scan Sam's ER letter into its database, so ER physicians would know exactly how to treat Sammy if he were brought into the hospital unconscious. Additionally, Nurse Iris came into Sam's room one day to provide us with a pamphlet showing how to buy car accessories for those with chronic medical conditions. I looked at the pamphlet. Amazing! I could buy bright orange sleeves that Velcroed around a car's seat belt. Each sleeve stated "MEDICAL INFORMATION" in bold, black letters. On the back of each was a zippered compartment where I could slide in a copy of Sam's ER instructions and cornstarch schedule. I remember that when we got home to New Jersey, I bought four of the neon wallets—two for Martin and me, one for Tee, and one for Sam's car. The kid couldn't even drive yet and certainly didn't have a car, but we would be ready for that day.

Does this all sound a bit obsessive? Since Sammy had been born, I had run on a rampant high alert. I had planned, ordered medical supplies, met with teachers, and reviewed his medical forms—all to be ready for "that day" when Sammy left our control. It was exhausting.

One year later, we headed to Gainesville again to be part of Dr. Weinstein's final study of nighttime cornstarch. In this study, the endocrinologist and his team fine-tuned dosing requirements for the new starch. Again, Sammy "lasted" eight hours on the new starch both nights. By this time, Sammy was five foot eleven. Before we'd get ready to leave the hospital for our day's fun and adventure, he'd go visit a patient's room, with Dr. Weinstein's permission. He'd normally visit a GSD baby or toddler, the parents often sitting by the bed in numb despair.

Sammy was a chatty guy. Within thirty minutes, the parents would learn that Sammy was a ninth grader. He was going to take driver's ed. He had been on the swim team. He had a girl named Samantha who liked him. He'd been on sleepovers. He'd been to camp. He was still working on his hovercraft. He had once eaten a roly-poly bug on a dare. His *mean* big brother threw cicadas on him two years ago.

Each time, we'd see hope creep into the parents' faces. Sammy symbolized a "normal" kid—if "normal" really exists in this world. I would talk the parents through steps that would help their child become more independent. Sammy and I tried to be Team GSD hope. Turns out that GSD hope is much like diabetes hope, Down syndrome hope, spina bifida hope.

When Sammy was a sophomore in college, the new cornstarch product launched—Glycosade, by Vitaflo USA. To this day, hundreds of individuals with GSD use this product to achieve something you and I take for granted: a good night's sleep. However, here's the irony of Sammy's beta-testing adventures: he can't use Glycosade because it makes his stomach hurt. So, he still takes regular cornstarch, every three hours, every day, every week, every month, every year.

***

A few months after our second testing session at the University of Florida hospital, I got an email from Dr. Weinstein. In addition to GSD 1a, his research team was studying GSD 1b. Would Sammy and I be available to go to the NIH in Bethesda, Maryland, to provide a blood sample during summer break? An anonymous GSD 1b patient would simultaneously provide a sample too. The blood work had to be drawn at the same time for effective testing and data storage. Dr. Weinstein and other scientists were attempting to determine differences in blood composition that might account for the additional difficulties incurred by type 1b patients.

Dr. Weinstein knew that Sammy was somewhat a science whiz kid. So, the endocrinologist provided us basic information on the differences between GSD 1a and b. Essentially, the enzyme deficiency in 1a is the glucose-6-phosphatase-α catalytic subunit, impacting the G6PC gene. In GSD 1b, however, the enzyme deficiency is the glucose-6-phosphate transporter, impacting a different gene. Both diseases are considered autosomal recessive and present themselves in the liver.[7] Type 1a occurs in 1/100,000 of the general population, impacting specifically the Ashkenazi Jewish, Mormon, Mexican, and Chinese heritages. On the other hand, 1b accounts for only 10 to 15 percent of all type 1 GSD cases. High-risk populations for 1b include Native Americans, Iranian Jews, and those of Italian heritage.[8]

Here's the rub, however. According to Dr. Weinstein, GSD

7. Borhane Annabi et al., "The Gene for Glycogen Storage Disease Type 1b Maps to Chromosome 11q23," *AJHG* 62, no. 2 (February 1998): 400–405, accessed March 13, 2020, https://doi.org/10.1086/301727.

8. Annabi et al., "Maps to Chromosome 11q23."

1b may appear clinically similar to 1a for many years. At some point, however, patients with 1b will develop neutropenia, which can cause numerous infections and fevers, much like a cancer survivor who has undergone chemo. GSD 1b patients also suffer from inflammatory bowel disease, resembling Crohn's.[9] In other words, the 1b patient must manage "typical" GSD conditions plus neutropenia and inflammatory bowel disease.

After I got the email from Dr. Weinstein, I snagged Sammy after school, luring him to the kitchen island with unbuttered popcorn. I showed him Dr. Weinstein's email and the information about GSD 1b patients.

"Jeez. They have it a lot worse than I do. Oh, my God." Sammy slid his hand, blue and grubby from art class, up through his curls.

"So, what do you think?"

"Can I do this before I start driver's ed? That's in late June."

"Sure. Let me call the NIH tomorrow. Dr. Weinstein has provided us a testing case number to refer to. He said something about paperwork we will need to fill out before we go."

When Dr. Weinstein said "paperwork," it was an understatement. Within a week of calling the NIH, I received a hefty packet in the mail. I dove into the pile of forms. I had to list my current address plus the three prior ones. Jobs, date of birth, social security number, parents' last names. The make and model of my car, as well as the license plate number. Countries outside the US the family had traveled to, and when. An official passport photo of myself and of Sammy. The NIH did not mess around.

In mid-June, Sammy and I drove three and a half hours to Bethesda to the massive NIH campus. We pulled up to the Gateway Center, stopping at the guardhouse.

"Hi!" I smiled at the guard, hoping my Kansas dimples

9. Chen and Weinstein, "Glycogen Storage Diseases," 51.

would let us breeze through quickly. We had to be in the lab in one hour, first dumping off our suitcases at the Children's Inn adjacent to the lab building.

The guard was not impressed by my Kansas dimples or fluttering of eyelashes. "Out of the car, please. Both of you." Two other guards appeared, along with a bomb-sniffing dog. Sammy and I stood, as directed, in a painted square about twenty feet away. A German shepherd circled the vehicle, sniffing intently for explosives, cocaine, and Uzis. He found nothing exciting, other than packages of snacks. One guard popped our trunk, took out the suitcases, and zipped them open, lifting our shorts and my pj's with a stick. The other guard walked around the car with a mirror attached to a pole, examining the car undercarriage for more explosive devices. Guard number one circled to the interior of my station wagon, zipped open Sammy's backpack, and took out boxes of Argo cornstarch and plastic containers with a mysterious white powder. He took them inside the guardhouse, scanning the containers and boxes with a gizmo much like we had seen at security at airports. Sure enough, we had no explosives, heroin, or cocaine. Just cornstarch. Lots of cornstarch.

Just a few minutes later, Sammy and I headed back to the lab building, up several floors, down more halls, and into a sterile waiting area. I felt like Sniff and Scurry in their race to find cheese in a maze.

After ten minutes in the phlebotomy lab, Sammy sauntered out, his blood drawn and mouth swabbed. Somewhere in the maze of laboratories nearby, a child with GSD 1b did the same thing. Both sets of parents signed paperwork that the genetic data of each child should go into databases at the NIH, the Children's Hospital of Philadelphia, the University of Florida, and Duke University. Both sets of parents prayed for productive research, for hope.

Sammy and I will never know exactly how his genetic

information benefited patients with GSD 1b. These patients can often manage the hypoglycemic issues of their condition, but the neutropenia and inflammatory bowel complications continue to plague them. However, as with many medical mysteries, scientists have made progress. In 2017, researchers at the NIH successfully used AAV-mediated gene therapy to restore GSD 1b mice that experienced fasting hypoglycemia.[10] In 2019, researchers led by Veiga da Cuntha published that GSD 1b neutropenia "could be treated by administration of kidney glucose transporter inhibitor (SGLT2 inhibitor)."[11] The hope and research continue.

Somewhere, amidst the cornstarch, the Mic-key button, the blood work, the syringes, the restricted diet, lies purpose. Sammy knows he has stepped forward to help others with GSD. I think back to story time with Sammy when he bored into my soul with his large, blue eyes, asking, "Why did God give me GSD?" Perhaps God knew that Sammy would help another child.

---

10. Fabienne Rajas, "Lessons from New Mouse Models of Glycogen Storage Disease Type 1a in Relation to the Time Course and Organ Specificity of the Disease," *Journal of Inherited Metabolic Disease* 38, no. 3 (May 2015): 521–527.
11. Rajas, "Lessons from New Mouse Models."

28

Mic-key Be Gone

"I want to get rid of it."

I was sitting next to Sammy at the kitchen bar, his backpack spewing out its usual contents of wadded-up homework and red tickets. Tee would be home after track practice, so I always seized this time to eat popcorn with Sammy, do a little English homework ("Mom, *The Yearling* stinks"), and catch up on his life.

"My new endocrine doc said that my growth is right on track. I'm fifteen and five foot eleven. But, the kids in gym class look at me funny with this Mic-key button."

My heart felt a slight pang. I remembered my middle school days of braces, glasses, and zits. I remembered how, in the locker room, *some* girls had cool turquoise bras and an awesome body to go into them. I remembered how, at the time, I did *not* have a cool turquoise bra *or* an awesome body. I just wanted to be like everyone else, because to be different in middle or high school was humiliating. Sammy had been fairly indifferent about his GSD condition thus far, but the Mic-key button . . . This was different. It was an outward sign that he was not the *same* as others.

"Okay, okay. I'll call the endocrinologist at the Children's Hospital. Now, Sammy, do you realize what this means when the Mic-key button is gone?"

"Yeah. I know. I'll have to get up in the night and mix up my cornstarch and gulp it down."

"Right. The rest of your life. No more Mom doing the dose through the Mic-key while you sleep. You'll have to do it. Every night. Even when you're tired."

"Mom, I can do it." Sam was dead serious.

"Okay, then."

The next day, I tracked down our endocrinologist.

"Actually," he said, "you can use the small syringe that comes with the Mic-key button. Remove the liquid from the balloon in the stomach and gently pull the button out. Clean the area three times a day, apply Vaseline, and keep a large square of gauze securely taped over it. The hole should begin to heal up in two to four weeks. It's about three millimeters in diameter, right?"

It didn't heal up. Sammy was a complicated guy.

About six weeks after Sammy had removed his Mic-key button, he was in GI surgery at the Children's Hospital of Philadelphia. The hole into his stomach was stitched shut. Within months, all that remained was a thumbnail smile of a scar. Mic-key was gone.

***

Time seemed to accelerate during the rest of Sammy's high school years. Meanwhile, Tee had gone off to Radford University in Virginia. The nine-hour drive to see him for parents' weekend had left Martin and me sobbing all the way back—it had been our first visit to see "the college boy." One day the following week, I even found myself sniveling into my shopping cart at the local ShopRite grocery. The separation was hard for us as parents, but Tee was in absolute heaven. Radford had the green lawns and redbrick buildings that glossy college brochures are made of. Tee was busy with business classes, tag football, girls, a fraternity, parties, and—did I say *girls*? Tee had been popular in high school, becoming a high-hurdles track star and attracting a number of "Joisey" girls. Now, at Radford, he was Mr. Social King and president of his fraternity.

I couldn't ever tell if Sammy missed Tee. Sammy took over our downstairs playroom, with neighbor kids coming daily to dominate a quick game of *Grand Theft Auto* before homework time. We filled one end of the small playroom with a complete set of pre-owned drums for Sam, including high hats, toms, and a cowbell. I remember standing a floor above in our kitchen, squishing hamburger, eggs, and onions through my fingers, preparing to create a good old Kansas meat loaf. Down below, Sammy would sit with his drum teacher, Mr. Caputo. The instructor had played with Bo Diddley, and boy, did it show. I could almost feel the air of excitement as Mr. Caputo would lean forward in his chair, encouraging Sammy, "Now, let's practice the double paradiddle! Then, the shuffle groove." Sammy would lay into his drums, making my red salt and pepper shakers dance along the kitchen countertop. The noise was deafening, yet the noise was great.

So, Sammy was fine without big brother Thomas. Thomas was flourishing at Radford, while Sammy flourished—torment-free from cicadas—in Pittstown.

***

More saints entered into Sammy's life when he was in high school.

Dr. Rittler taught American History, British History, and Comparative World Cultures at Sam's school. His wife, Jane, taught A/P English. She caught on in a New York minute that Sammy was not actually reading the assigned novels. Sam was smart, of course. He'd read the first five chapters of each book, and CliffsNotes-it through the rest. His footnotes in his papers only ranged from chapters one through five.

Sammy, a good writer, got a C on his first paper.

"Do you find nothing worthy to footnote in the rest of *The Rule of the Bone*?" Mrs. Rittler pinned Sammy to his chair one day with a deadly stare, while the other seven students smirked.

"Uh . . . uh . . . uh." The smooth-talking Sammy was convicted. Amazingly, he began to read each of the remaining five novels of the course. And the goof-off student found he loved reading.

Dr. Rittler opened Sam's eyes in his class on Comparative World Cultures. Sam, along with his other classmates, had known little injustice in fifteen years of middle-class whiteness. Their worst battles involved "unfair" coaches or "mean" teachers who objected to paper airplanes sailing through the air. Dr. Rittler, however, taught the kids about atrocities conducted by the "good guys" during the Bosnian War. He dealt with the Tungchow mutiny, the Bodo League massacre, and the ethnic cleansing of Circassia. Sammy, a growing conspiracy-theory lover, became enraged as he learned about atrocities in Latin America, mostly sponsored by the US government at the behest of the boards of directors of various fruit companies. He, fellow students, and Dr. Rittler gathered with others to protest the killings in Darfur. Sammy picketed against the policies at Wal-Mart that hedged health benefits. I was thrilled. In the sea of apathetic teens that cared only about the next party, Sammy became engaged and morphed from a class clown to a passionate student. I owe all to Dr. and Mrs. Rittler and others who nudged and encouraged Sam. As a Congolese priest friend of ours says, "You can't pick up a nut with one finger." Raising a child is indeed a team effort. It's a long, massive effort.

***

At the end of each academic year, Sammy's school would conduct two full days of final exams, with each subject encompassing two hours. At the end of final exams, the students were given an opportunity to take two weeks of optional, outside-of-class learning. Ninth graders had to stay locally instead of travel, so, of course, Sam took improvisation. The "Joisey" cab driver in him longed for more expression. At the end of his tenth-grade year, Sammy was given the opportunity to travel with teachers and classmates to Israel.

"I really want to go! Dr. Rittler and his wife will be going with us. Twelve of us will be selected to go for the nine-day journey." What Sammy neglected to tell me was that the trip would include areas near the bombings at the Gaza Strip and the West Bank. The Gaza War had been in our news a lot in 2008. I had seen bloody battles on television between the Palestinian paramilitary groups and the Israel Defense Forces. A class trip to an area where rockets blew up targets, soldiers, and civilians? A scary area.

Martin and I have always believed that at least half of a person's education occurs outside the classroom. We wanted both of our sons to know more than just the immediate bubble surrounding their lives. But nine days in Israel. Tel Aviv was fifty-seven hundred miles away and a six-hour time difference. Israel was a high-tech country, but also a country with political and spiritual tensions. We didn't know the country's hospitals or the doctors. This was no little jaunt to Bryn Mawr, but I was determined that Sammy would have opportunities similar to his classmates. Independence for Sammy was a journey—sometimes just a step a day. But this was a massive stride.

Martin and I met with Dr. Rittler and Mrs. Rittler, much like we had done with Mrs. Meeks at Bryn Mawr. We reviewed Sam's ER letter and cornstarch schedule. We discussed nearby hospitals where the group would be staying in Israel, should Sammy get the stomach flu. We detailed food restrictions. The Rittlers were "on"; Martin and I began gathering supplies, updating medical forms, and checking Sammy's vaccinations. A lawyer friend had advised us on a power of attorney for medical care, which had to be drafted, signed, and stamped by a notary public. Apparently, some hospitals and medical practices would not admit a minor child if not accompanied by a parent or guardian. Martin and I would take no chances regarding this trip to Israel.

Of course, the differences between Israel and Bryn Mawr are huge. For the trip to Israel, we had figured out, with Dr. Rittler's assistance, how close the various hospitals were at each point of the itinerary, obtaining their addresses and telephone numbers for the Rittlers, Sammy, and us. Fortunately, the sponsors had a mobile phone with international calling abilities. Equally important, we had to make sure Sammy had a box of Argo cornstarch for each day he would be gone, plus several more in case of accidental spillage.

The average traveler doesn't know that Argo cornstarch can't be purchased in a typical grocery store in Israel, or in Britain, Ireland, or Martinique, for that matter. Sometimes you can find "corn flour," but structurally, it's not the same; it fails to keep blood sugar up adequately. Sometimes, you're lucky and can find tapioca starch, which is a good substitute for Argo. Also, the average traveler doesn't know how nervous the TSA becomes when a teen shows up in security with small bottles of white powder, Citrucel, and multiple boxes of Argo. It's a showstopper, GSD travel letter or no travel letter. To ease the potential panic at the airport, we always insisted that Sammy get a decent haircut before travel and wear a collared polo shirt and dockers. It wasn't the time to look scruffy. It was sad but true; stereotyping was alive and well. We never knew when Sammy might have to talk his way out of a situation.

Our son contacted several of his buddies going on the same flight to Israel. Sure, they could also carry several boxes of Argo apiece in their backpacks. All told, fourteen boxes would travel to Israel from Newark. I knew the TSA would get suspicious seeing the massive amounts of white powder making its way to Tel Aviv. Ironically, when Sam waived his GSD travel letter under one TSA worker's nose, the man snorted impatiently and shoved the letter aside. Instead, he began methodically wanding each plastic jar of cornstarch, each jar of Citrucel, and each box of Argo. The airport security line backed up like a clogged pipe, as the thorough guard also pulled out catheter tip syringes, Imodium tablets, and Zofran. He dumped packages of crackers and popcorn into a blue plastic TSA bin. With an abrupt nod and a push of the bin, the guard finally sent Sammy through security. I remember Martin and I stood behind rope barriers, seeing our baby greet his classmates and begin to distribute his cornstarch stash. With a quick turn back to us and a smile, Sammy disappeared into the mass of people, and out of our control.

Sam and his buddies were scattered throughout the crowded El Al flight. Most of the passengers were Hasidic Jews. During the long flight, the passengers repeated the Tefillot (prayers) twice. Sammy, as he told me later, remembered being antsy, attempting to fold his long legs into the cramped seating space. He read a bit of *Fear and Loathing in Las Vegas* and dug around his backpack for snacks. He drifted off to sleep periodically, only to be awakened by the soft murmuring periodically resonating through the plane. He arrived in Tel Aviv early in the morning, bleary-eyed from little sleep and multiple time zones.

Normally, I'd expect the sponsors to let the kids regroup the first morning. After all, they'd been on a long overnight flight from Newark, New Jersey. But no. That morning, sponsors led the group on a rigorous bicycle ride through Masada National Park. Somehow, Sam made it through the ride, feeling sick and exhausted from little sleep and sketchy food. Some of the more rambunctious kids even decided to hike to the top of the Masada fortress at 5:00 a.m. the next day. Sam decided to sleep in a bit, reckoning that a *sunset* would look just as good as a *sunrise*, right?

However, Sam told us when he got home that his time in Israel was magical. In addition to Masada, Dr. Rittler's group visited the Baha'i Gardens and the Sea of Galilee. In the cities, the bell towers rang daily with the call to worship for the Jews, the Muslims, the Christians, and the Druze. Sammy's travel group feasted on hummus and tahini—a far cry from our baked chicken *à la Aunt Alice* at home. I found out later that the highlight of the trip was the Ein Gedi Reserve, a beautiful hiking and swimming spot in the middle of the Judean desert. "Mom, our group hiked along the oasis trails to this waterfall. In the middle of the desert! It was huge, and we even got to see some old ruins along the way. I saw some poplar trees by the side of the lake, just like in our backyard in Kansas. I knew I wasn't in Kansas anymore. But I'll tell you—if I see one more plate of hummus . . ."

"Did you click your ruby slippers together to get back home?" I teased.

"Oh, Mom." Eye roll. Eye roll. I had missed my teen with the attitude. Most importantly, my son had managed his GSD well on the trip, despite different time schedules, food, climate, and activities. Sammy came back exhausted, but alive and determined that GSD, that ever-present companion, would not hold him back.

29

Joe College

It seemed like I had just quit sniveling over Tee's absence, yet we were about to launch child number two into college. How could that be? The boys were only six years apart. College. The halls of academia, but more likely, the halls of little sleep. Of fraternities. Of drinking. Of temptations galore. Of frightening independence. Of necessary independence.

Dr. Rittler's influence was ever present as Sammy applied for various colleges. Would it be Dickinson College, Franklin & Marshall, or the University of North Carolina? Duke? Nope. He had good grades but not good enough for Duke. Perhaps American University or George Washington University? Sammy was intent on studying international relations, with an eye toward grad school, he told us one night at dinner. A rainbow of lettuce, salsa, and refried beans lay scattered around Sammy's plate, a death knell from his tacos.

Sammy and I looked at colleges, while Martin worked

away, preparing for the next tuition blast. Sammy and I would go on college tours, absorb the admissions hype, then hang in any student common area we could find.

"Yeah. The kids at Franklin & Marshall look pretty serious." We sat at a picnic table in the commons area, sipping sugar-free lemonade and eating Cheetos. Sam was right! The students walked to and from class, quiet, heads down. The mom in me wondered, *Is that a bad thing?*

"Well, maybe they're here, uh, to study?" I said in my most motherly tone.

I got my third eye roll of the day. It was a banner day for being an annoying mom.

After all the tours, forms, essays, interviewing, testing, and epic gnashing of teeth, it was down to two universities: George Washington University in DC or the University of Delaware in Newark. George Washington was a city school with a powerhouse international relations department and significant government connections. On the other hand, U Del had wide, green lawns; redbrick buildings with ivy; and, most importantly, *more cute girls than George Washington.* "I know that there are at least thirty percent more cute girls at U Del!" Sam told me several times on our trip home from Delaware. Had he been making a tally on his cell phone? Brunette? Check. Blonde? Check. Redhead? Check.

"I don't know what to do!" Sammy would wail to me five times daily after the college visits. "GW has all kinds of government ties that might be helpful to me in my future career or maybe law school. But U Del *looks* like a college is supposed to look. The kids seem to be happy and connecting with each other. There are fraternities, and I saw some blondes. . . ."

Uh-oh. The mom in me jumped into high alert. *Fraternities. Girls. Drinking. Sleeping through the cornstarch dose. Hospital ER. Liver adenomas the size of a lemon.* My mind zipped from *A* to *Z* with dizzying speed.

"Well, I'm going upstairs to take a shower and think on it," he said. I had never heard of thinking in the shower, but it was close to singing, right? Within two minutes, I heard the soft whoosh of water above me, followed by a sharp clunk of the soap hitting the shower floor, followed by a loud "arghhhhhhh." More thunks of soap hitting the floor and then the frustrated slap-slap-slap of flip-flops. Apparently, Sam was throwing soap and thinking about his college selection.

He came into the kitchen minutes later slightly damp, sporting only his plaid boxers. I pretended to be busy looking over an expense report, tallying columns of numbers for a part-time job I had. "I've decided," Sam announced. *Good thing,* I thought. The deadline to pay by credit card was *tonight,* at midnight. Nothing like taking it down to the wire.

"It's going to be U Del. I have to learn but have fun at the same time." Sam pulled raw carrots and ranch dip out of the fridge and began munching. Contemplating in the shower apparently made a person ravenous. Or maybe it was just being eighteen.

"You know, Sam, I lived at home my first year of college and was absolutely miserable. It was for financial reasons, you see. But I worked hard the next summer and made enough money to live on campus my sophomore year. Strangely enough, my fun level went up one hundred percent, and my grades went up to all As. Play hard, work hard, as they say. But in your case, don't play *too* hard. . . ."

I got yet another eye roll for my efforts and dug out my credit card to phone in the tuition deposit. The card would soon be burning and continue to flame brightly each semester.

***

I wish I could report that Sam's college years were uneventful, but of course, they weren't.

Sam's dorm roommate and soon-to-be-best-bud at U Del was dark-haired Cody, a kid from a speck of a town called Magnolia, Delaware. Cody had black-fringed eyes and a slow drawl that belied his incredible intelligence.

We were in the dorm room amidst piles of school supplies, computer cables, and sort-of-clean clothes. "Uh. Cody. I wanted to let you know about these containers of white powder that you'll be seeing here on Sam's bookcase. Well, it's not cocaine." I was busy with notebooks and file folders while Martin vacuumed. I grinned inwardly at my feeble attempt at a joke, continuing to explain Sammy's condition to Cody.

"It's no problem. I'm cool with it. Hey, looks like you could use some help with that futon." Cody leaned back in his desk chair and eyed a jumble of parts on the dorm-room floor.

Cody was right. Martin and I, sporting six degrees combined, had thirty parts of a futon frame scattered around the doom floor. It was a hopeless mess of boards, bolts, and nuts, but Cody, the budding engineering major, dragged out his blue toolbox and began to assemble the futon. I didn't know what kind of kid brought a full-fledged toolbox to college, but I did know this. Cody was smart and patient—an all-around good guy with four—count 'em—four types of wrenches.

Within weeks, Cody and Sammy pledged a fraternity and jumped into coursework. They also jumped into parties and girls. Most importantly, Sammy renewed his passion for improvisation. He became a member of the campus group called the Riot Act, practicing four nights a week. Somehow, amidst all the frantic activity, Sammy did study, double majoring in international relations and economics. His minor was philosophy, which meant that, over the next three years, he and I would have interesting conversations on the Copenhagen concept or determinism and freedom in society. I loved these exchanges with Sammy and would scurry to Wikipedia afterward to look up what the heck we had been discussing.

30

Licking the Taj Mahal

U Del had a trimester system, which meant that the students had the entire month of January to work or do a short travel-abroad class. Now, I had never traveled abroad in college—that was just for rich kids. Instead, I worked between terms at the campus instructional media department, cleaning sixteen-millimeter films with toxic chemicals and wheeling around carts precariously loaded with projectors and clunky monitors.

Sammy arrived home for fall break his freshman year at U Del. Nearly breathless, he burst in the door, hugged me, and promptly handed me a mesh clothes hamper. In a moment of madness the prior week, I had volunteered to do laundry, since Sam had been busy studying for midterms and performing improv. He was probably also making tallies of blondes, red-heads, and brunettes on his cell phone.

I gave Sam a massive mom hug back as he lugged the mesh container into our laundry room. I pulled out two white tee shirts. Within seconds, polka-dot boxers and ragged jeans sprang out of the container, sending up a sweaty, college-boy smell with them. I turned my head, pulling out an item at a time with my thumb and forefinger. One load of laundry, washed twice. A second load, washed twice. A third load. A fourth. A fifth. As it turned out, Sammy had done no laundry for two months. Zip. Nada. I guess he was too busy performing with the Riot Act and thinking about metaphysics. Apparently, clean boxers were a plebian detail of life. After all, you could get three wearings out of each pair: front to back, back to front, and inside out. And—there was always commando.

Sam followed me into the laundry room, impervious to the wafting stink. "Mom! You'll never guess what I can do this January for a class! U Del offers a January travel-abroad class. It's offered by Dr. Gitu Barua, a professor of Indian literature. We would travel for twenty-five days, going to Assam, Agra, Goa . . . uh, I forget the other states. It would be so cool. We would get to see the Taj Mahal, the Amber Palace, and the Agra Fort. We would study Indian literature, which has been totally ignored in our culture."

Sammy rolled this information off his tongue as casually as if he were driving down the street to Wal-Mart to buy sneakers. As a kid from Kansas, how did he know about India?

Sam took a deep breath and began a forward verbal launch. "This would be so good for my international relations major at U Del. I've got to start building my résumé now."

I had to hand it to Sam. He was a smooth talker. I stood in the laundry room, a bit stunned. India? I sat down at the tiny table in the corner of the room and Googled rapidly. India. About eighty-two hundred miles away. Over one billion people. Oh . . . over nine hours' time difference. Holy smokes.

The Kansan/mom/perfectionist/worrier started thinking about germs. Real germs. I had read somewhere that India had more than its share of germs. I Googled some more, and there it was: "India has one of the world's highest number of bacterial infections; tuberculosis, cholera, typhoid, pneumonia and a host of them. In fact, the country has the highest number of tuberculosis patients in the world, accounting for one-fourth of all TB patients in the world. Multidrug-resistant (MDR) and extensively drug-resistant (XDR) tuberculosis cases are increasingly reported."[1] I pushed back from my table, feeling pretty sick in my heart. Multidrug-resistant cases?

"I don't know, Sam," I said, rubbing my forehead with anxiety. "Look at this data. If you get any stomach issues and can't get to a hospital within about two hours . . ."

"Mom! Mom!" Sam revved up like an encyclopedia salesman. "We're staying all over India, but with families that *own* schools. They're 'comfortable,' as you and Dad like to say. Their houses will be much nicer than ours. They have servants and doctors and hospitals there. Dr. Barua grew up in India and went to undergrad there. *Are you seriously going to keep me at home the next forty years and tuck me under your arm?*"

"Maybe." I smiled weakly at Sam, knowing that every fiber in my body wanted to protect him and, yes, tuck him under my arm forever. Our family had been through so much, so much. Yes, walking to independence was good, vital; but this India trip scared me to my core.

***

It wasn't until we got pages and pages of data about the month in India that I began to relax. Just a tiny bit.

Martin and I faced this dilemma: Just how much do you "let go" of a child with a chronic condition? Sure, Sammy had navigated his time in Israel well as a high schooler. He had gone

1. Sapna Chhabra, "India Harbors Superbugs Everywhere—Do We Care?," *Research Matters*, April 13, 2018, https://researchmatters.in/news/india-harbors-superbugs-everywhere-%E2%80%93-do-we-care.

the next year to Japan for nine days with a class group. Both trips went by without incident. But the stakes were higher for the trip to India. Farther away. Longer. Scarier. Would I have let Tee go on such a trip? Were we being proactive in letting Sam take such a huge step to independence? Or were we just being irresponsible parents?

The research I had read so far about parenting chronically ill children wasn't helpful. Nearly all of it was framed in terms of parenting a five-year-old. Have Johnny set the table or throw his toys into the playroom bin. Here's the thing. My "child" was nineteen years old and six feet tall, standing in my laundry room and begging to go to India—eighty-two hundred miles away. My "child" lived life just hours from death, if events turned sour.

Despite all this, some helpful suggestions exist (even after reminders of how primary caregivers may find it difficult to adapt to a new role). The University of Michigan Health System website provides additional information to guide me through Sammy's development. For example, our family must stay involved with Sammy; give information; plan for procedures; give him choices, support his friendships; be hopeful; listen; teach coping skills; stay organized; be aware of the risks unique to Sam's illness.[2] It's all great advice, but I'd challenge any parent to be able to do all this perfectly. The problem is, when your chronically ill child is a flesh-and-blood Sammy, all you want to do is hug him, throw out the scholarly articles, and never, never let go. Your heart can hardly take it. If you nearly lose him one more time . . .

But we decided to let Sam go to India. I do remember our family's decision process. Our questions looked something like this:

---

2. University of Michigan Health System, accessed September 1, 2020, http://www.med.umich.edu/yourchild/topics/chronic.htm (site discontinued).

- How are Sam's general health and GSD control?
- How well is he trained to manage his day-to-day health?
- Is Sam a responsible individual, laundry aside?
- How does he conduct himself in the emergency room and at doctor's appointments?
- How has Sam handled his previous travel?
- Has he been responsible and health conscious at college the last two months? What are his grades?
- How trustworthy are the faculty sponsors on the trip to India?
- Are hospitals available near every point in the itinerary?
- Can Sam get a working cell phone once he lands in India?
- What are the ramifications of the multiple vaccinations required?
- Can Sam learn and follow explicitly his many food restrictions in India?
- Can we get students to help Sam lug thirty-five boxes of cornstarch to and around India?
- Would we have let Tee take such a trip? How important is brotherly equality in the family?

As always, the dust settled after many discussions. Sammy would go to study in India with Dr. Barua. After all, we had let Tee go on a school trip to Peru when he was twelve. Tee had to dodge snakes and spiders on his trip, as he and his classmates stayed in a lodge near the tree line in Machu Picchu. Tee came back home with an evil-looking, two-foot machete as well as a carved blowgun. Ironically, airport security had allowed him to put his machete in the overhead compartment of the airplane, as long as the weapon was securely wrapped in newspaper. Who knew that newspaper was an effective anti-terrorist device years ago?

"Sam, if you want to do this, you must obtain the name of a hospital for each location on the itinerary in India. Dr. Barua has this information, I'm sure. You will also need to meet with her in November to go through all your medical forms. This week, please call Dr. Rushton to get a list of vaccinations needed for your trip, and I will schedule them. We probably need to start on some shots this week. This is all your responsibility."

Back when Sam was in high school, we had done some of the preparatory work for his camps or trips, but now, he was a college student. He had to step up. It wouldn't be that long before he was out working, we hoped. Another step. More responsibility. More independence.

Flash forward. Sammy got listings of hospitals and phone numbers for his travels, as well as names of host families in India and phone numbers. He endured vaccinations for hepatitis A, hepatitis B, typhoid, cholera, yellow fever, Japanese encephalitis, rabies, meningitis, polio, MMR, Tdap, pneumonia, and influenza. The kid became a human pincushion. While Sam was enduring multiple shots, we were navigating the painful visa application process. It seemed that India, like the NIH, wanted every vestige of information about us.

***

It was midmorning at the Newark airport. Ten kids gathered with Dr. Barua, ready to go through airport security to board a United Airlines flight. The kids would be airborne for about fifteen hours, barreling through several time zones. During this time, Sam would have to manage numerous small snacks and his cornstarch, measured out to last four hours apiece. Once the kids landed, the group would buy cell phones in the airport.

I met all the students in the group, along with Dr. Barua. True to his word, Sam had talked to each one about his cornstarch and medical condition. No big deal. Each kid put three boxes of Argo in a backpack while Sam toted five. I gave Sam what I hoped was a non-mushy-gooshy hug as the group prepared to go through security.

"Don't forget to buy water once you go through! Use your antibacterial wipes! Call me! Protect your passport. Don't drink the water in India. Have—"

"Okay, Janet." My husband put a restraining hand on my shoulder, but I think I heard a little quiver in his voice. "Sam's got this."

I felt excitement for Sam. What would he see and experience? And I also felt real dread—that sick-in-the-heart feeling. My baby was going to be far, far away—completely away from my ability to help him. *What did Martin and I just do here?*

In the days ahead, my heart simply raced when Sammy called us.

"Mom, India is full of the most beautiful sights in the world and also the most heart-wrenching." Sam went on to tell us of shanties built in the road medians and the exotic, crowded spice markets rich with the scent of garam masala and cumin. "I never forget I'm in India," he would tell us excitedly on the phone. "And guess what! We go to the Taj Mahal tomorrow."

Sometimes, four or five days crept by before I heard from Sam, because certain states in India did not permit cell phone contact with the US. During those days, I prayed often, thinking back to the poem "Footprints" that carried me years ago. I knew from the itinerary which state Sam was in on which day, but it was just a name for me. I was a Kansas girl and not well traveled. During Sam's trip, I was being tested on both faith and on letting go. Both concepts were uncomfortable for me, so you could say as Sam was growing and experiencing, so was I.

Reuniting with the group at the end of twenty-five days was exhilarating. I'd never seen a group of kids so excited yet so bedraggled.

Over the next two weeks, Martin and I heard more and more stories about India. There was the time when Sam and another student were heading back from a spice market to their group, only to be chased by a pack of wild dogs. There were occasions when Sam would be staying with a "comfortable" family, only to be confused and upset by the extreme deference of the servants. In the Hayles family, we did our own cleaning, our own yard work, our own home repairs. Sam had never seen a caste system in operation before, and it disturbed him greatly. Our son had always talked to everyone everywhere anytime about everything, yet the servants in the comfortable Indian families would look down quietly when Sam would begin to chat. That understanding of the caste system in itself was worth the entire price of a college education. Sammy was beginning to whiff the scent of social inequality.

I also found out after Sam's return what had happened at the Taj Mahal. He and two others had sneaked around the reflection pond to one side of the monument. They had all stuck their tongues out, licking the ivory-white marble of the sacred mausoleum.

"Why?" I exploded when I heard this distressing tidbit of news. "Why would you have done something silly like this? Talk about picking up germs. And it's a *sacred* shrine!"

"Well, we figured that no one in history would have licked the outside wall of the Taj Mahal. It opened in 1648, and we were the first to do this!"

Perhaps there had been no one this foolish visiting the Taj Mahal since 1648. Doubt crept into my heart. Was Sammy truly mature enough to take on other trips? Seriously. Licking the Taj Mahal. At this point, I wanted my son to go nowhere else.

The last bombshell Sam dropped on us was that he had been sick in India. Sick! I hadn't known about it.

Apparently, Sam had been staying with one of the many families on the itinerary that owned a school. In fact, one of the sons became friends with Sam, giving him a designer scarf that cost more than my winter coat. At any rate, on day three with the family, Sam began to feel feverish and achy. The family called their doctor, who came out, examined Sam, and gave him a round of antibiotics. Within two days, fortunately, Sam rallied and was able to move on with the group. When he got home, he gave me the physician's receipt for services. The house call plus antibiotics equated to sixteen US dollars.

We will never know what "bug" Sam caught. The blessing was that he got home safely, with a lifetime of adventures, his eyes wide-open.

31

Tesorería General de la República

Sam's sophomore year rolled along smoothly. Schoolwork, improv, and fraternity obligations filled the days. In mid-October, Sam started conspiring for his upcoming January course. By this time, he was knee-deep in international relations and economics courses.

Sam burst into the house at fall break, this time *without* lugging a loaded laundry bag. Hmmmm. Could this be maturity in the works? Or did a mountainous pile of laundry exist back in Newark, Delaware?

At the table that night, Sam was full of stories about his roommate, Cody, who pulled all-night study sessions before tests and still got good grades. And why could Cody eat fries and drink Cokes and not get fat? Then there was the incident of a college kid caught by the police at the intersection of Main and Chapel streets in Newark. The problem was that he had only his boxers on and *may* have been inebriated. Martin and

I listened intently. The wild stories made us want to go back to college, except we'd both have to be in bed by ten to make it through the next day.

"Anyways, guys, here's what I found out about this winter break."

"*Anyway,* Sam. The word is *anyway.*"

"Whatever. There's an organization called World Wide Chile that helps students find internships in Chile and also shows them around the country. I could work for a month in Santiago, Chile, for their treasury department. I would be the first American intern to do that. Ever—ever! Wouldn't this be a great work experience to help me get my first job? And if I decide to go to law school, wouldn't this experience be a selling point?" Sammy, always the marketing man. His blue eyes, now behind navy frames, blazed with intensity.

Martin and I pushed our chicken Caesar around, stalling for time. World Wide Chile did sound intriguing as a brief experience in international work. And law school? This was the second time we'd heard about this plan. More big steps for Sam, more miles of separation, more independence. Wasn't that what we as parents had been working for?

I got to Googling again. Santiago. Fifty-one hundred miles from the Newark airport, give or take. A decently high standard of living. A volatile history. And then I probed Sam further: he would be with a group of other students interning various places in Santiago. The group had a sponsor who would organize cultural gatherings on weekends. Sam would stay with a host family and get food there. He could walk from his lodgings to his place of work during the month of January.

Planning for Chile was like planning for India, only there were fewer shots involved.

We had our medical checklists down cold. The dilemma of *this* trip was the cornstarch. Sam was traveling independently from Newark airport, meeting up at his host family's home in

Santiago via cab. That meant thirty-five boxes of cornstarch traveling with him. After some pondering, Sam came up with the solution. He'd have one large suitcase full of work shirts, khakis, and shorts, and an equally large suitcase of Argo. Add a computer bag. Add his backpack full of water, cornstarch containers, and snacks for fifteen hours. It would work, as long as both suitcases arrived with Sam in Santiago. What would happen if the suitcase with the Argo became lost? Sam could only carry five boxes in his backpack—and that would last him five days. He was fairly certain that packages from the US to Chile typically got waylaid by CorreosChile, the postal service. Then what? Then what?

One day, I sat down at my computer, arranging airfare for Sammy's big internship. It was all pricey, but finally, I found a decent fare on Continental Airlines to Santiago. Sam would fly from Newark to Haiti to Panama City to Santiago. A lot of transfers, but hey—it was affordable, and it was Continental Airlines. A big, stable company.

About twenty hours after Sam departed Newark, we got a call from him: he had landed in Santiago and had bought a temporary cell phone. He sounded shaken and rolled into a rant.

"Mom, don't ever have me fly again to Haiti!" I could hear a quiver in Sam's voice. "I'm not coming home that way. You've gotta check the flights back. I'm not doing it. You won't believe this. When we landed in Haiti, the airline officials made us get off the plane, totally leave the terminal, and walk around outside—outside, Mom!—to another terminal with all of our luggage. We had to go through security again. I walked out of the terminal and onto the tarmac, and then, presto. A man grabbed my suitcases and wouldn't let go without me giving him forty dollars. I mean, I had *two* huge suitcases, my computer bag, *and* my backpack. Then, as I was approaching the front of the airport, it happened again with a different man.

It was a bad situation." I could hear Sam inhale with agitation and fear.

"Oh, my God!" I could picture Sam, bogged down with baggage and trying to ward off people intent on "helping" him with his luggage. "Well, somehow you got out of this. What did you do?" I could feel the sickness of anxiety rising, bubbling up through my esophagus. What horrible situation had I put Sammy into?

I had never dreamed that Sam would be forced to exit one terminal in Haiti, only to battle his way into the second one. I felt terrible. How had I assumed flying would be the same everywhere? Thank goodness Sam was a daunting six foot two by his sophomore year. That didn't hurt a bit.

"Then, Mom." Another shaky inhalation. "When I got to security in the second terminal in Haiti, the guards gave me crap about having a whole suitcase full of Argo cornstarch."

"Maybe they thought you would be doing a lot of baking." My joke was wasted on Sam.

"I couldn't even talk to the guards, because I don't know Haitian Creole. I showed them my travel letter, and they just shoved it back at me. These were big, burly dudes with Berettas."

"How'd you get through? Did you know anyone else in line?" My anxiety rose and kept bubbling, like a caustic acid.

"Well, on the flight over, I sat next to a young doctor who flies to Haiti each year for a volunteer medical clinic. Thank goodness—she saw the ruckus and came forward to explain to the guards. I got through. But I'm just sayin', I'm never goin' . . ."

"I'm so sorry, Sam. I had no clue that you would have to go through with this experience. Such a good reaction and thinking on your part! I'll check the return flights when I get off the phone."

I tried to maintain my motherly calmness on the phone, but when I hung up, I melted into an emotional puddle. Sammy could have been kidnapped. He could have been robbed and stripped of all his money, his clothes, his medication. *What* would Martin and I have done? I think we all have times where the consequences of an event are just too horrible to wrap your head around. It's like a dark place in your brain, a sick place in your heart.

Needless to say, Sammy flew back home a different way.

***

Sammy made it to his host family in Santiago, a woman with a teen-aged son at home. Sam soon found out that the woman never really cooked; all he could find in the refrigerator was an occasional pastel de choclo—a corn casserole with meat. Sometimes, he'd spot an empanada. The problem was, most of the food in the home contained wheat, cheese, and rather greasy meat—absolutely nothing that Sammy could eat. Sam would take to wandering the street food stands after work, picking up items he could eat for breakfast or pack for lunch. Sometimes it was raw carrots or roasted chicken. He made do.

"TGR: Tesorería General de la República." The gold lettering across the front of the building was formal, impressive. I found out one phone call later that the treasury building sat near the presidential palace called La Moneda. The palace had been stormed when Augusto Pinochet took over Chile in a 1973 coup. Former president Salvador Allende was overthrown, and civilian rule ended.

"I'd walk to the treasury building and see bullet holes in the side of the palace," Sam told me during one phone call. "Legend has it those bullets were from Pinochet's troops. It's pretty cool to walk to work and see history."

"Tell me what your internship is like." It had only been

three days, but I was so excited for this opportunity for Sam. I had never been to South America. We saved our dollars for Tee and Sam to travel and learn.

"Well, the Tesorería is kind of like the US IRS. I'm working in the tax collection section. I create legal files regarding tax collection and update records. The job is really kind of like glorified data entry. My boss is really cool, though. He's an attorney and can speak some English."

"Are the others in the office pretty friendly?"

"They don't speak English. I remember some Spanish from high school, but not much. After work, I usually walk to a nearby bodega and get food. I've found shops where I can buy children's books in Spanish. My favorite is *My Name Is Gabriela*. Well, it's written for an eight-year-old, but I can teach myself more Spanish that way at night."

So, Sam was essentially reading a first-grade Tip primer and working for the Chilean IRS. Not a bad gig. By the end of January, Sam could speak hesitating Spanish to fellow workers in the office. By the following January, he had been invited again for a return internship. *Sammy era un tipo con suerte. Sammy was a lucky guy.* For once, he was lucky.

32

Five Steps Backward

During Sam's senior year in college, I started getting anxious phone calls from him. He was noticing tingling in his extremities and all over his skin. Headaches. Brain fog. GI issues. Tiredness. Rashes. You name it. Yes, he'd been to his doctor in Newark. No, she couldn't find anything wrong. Blood work normal. Blood pressure normal. No arrhythmia. Lungs were clear. Good oxygen intake. Sam got kicked down the line as a "whiner" to a GI specialist nearby. Meanwhile, Sam's symptoms swelled and diminished with no apparent pattern. *Something was wrong with my baby.*

Despite the growing storm of physical ailments, Sam graduated from U Del magna cum laude, only .001 of a point away from summa cum laude. As a mother, it was all I could do not to put a banner across the front of our house. In May, he came to his new home in Chapel Hill, North Carolina. Martin and I had moved there for retirement in 2013 when Sam became a senior. We loved New Jersey, but the property taxes made us choke. At any rate, Mr. U Del graduate took a class that summer and worked near the University of North Carolina campus at 'Sup Dog, bussing tables and wiping up pools of beer. Sammy had also applied at Borders Books, deeming that would be more "fun" since he was an avid reader. However, he committed what I call a Career Limiting Move, or CLM. In other words, on the way to the interview, Sam was running late. So, what was his plan of action? Cut off that white Buick to his left and screech into a parking spot right in front of Borders. During Sam's interview, the manager recognized Sam as the cocky young man who had just cut her off as she, too, was trying to park. Needless to say, the interview was over quickly. Mr. Sam was relegated to 'Sup Dog.

***

One beautiful Carolina evening in June, Sam, Martin, and I sat out on our tiny screened-in porch, taking in the sixty-foot pine trees. Martin and I sipped a goblet of Chardonnay that cast off a golden light—I remember holding the glass up and admiring the glint. Sam sipped a Diet Coke, his clothing still grubby and spotted from running the 'Sup Dog dishwasher.

"I'm gonna have hot dog under my nails forever!" he moaned. "I'm losing *my soul* at 'Sup Dog."

Martin and I reminded Sam that we had both worked at small-time drugstore cafés. We, too, had washed dishes, scraped off the blackened café grill, and made cherry phosphates and peanut hickeys. We had both walked two miles in the snow to get to work. Our tips were dimes and quarters. I used to wear a hairnet at the soda fountain where I worked, looking like Gladys Ormphby on *Laugh-In*. Martin and I had lost our souls working, too, but it was character building.

Sam listened to "Tough Times Parental Lecture 101" with

glazed eyes of boredom. Parental lecture aside, the three of us hammered out a plan for fall. Sam jotted down the list:

- Study for the LSAT and attend Princeton Review classes
- Continue losing my soul at 'Sup Dog
- Take another improv class or two
- Handle my laundry and wash dishes at Chez Hayles
- Help Mom tutor at a nearby Latino community

Sam's spring semester would be at Malaca Instituto in Málaga, Spain. Grandma B. had sent Sammy a nice check for graduation, specifying that it had to be spent on education. Then there were checks from Aunt Carol, Cousin Gerri, and Grandma Mae. We could do this. Spanish fluency and international relations? It did make sense as a next-step career plan.

So, the plan for life was on. Except it wasn't.

***

As summer 2014 progressed into fall, Sam's condition worsened, with headaches, nausea, and GI symptoms smacking him without reason. We wedged medical appointments between 'Sup Dog and LSAT classes. We had Sammy's internist mystified. In fact, we had specialists in neurology, infectious diseases, rheumatology, dermatology, and gastroenterology mystified. Sam was tested for Lyme disease, the Epstein-Barr virus, mono, low vitamin D levels, chronic fatigue syndrome, fibromyalgia, Sjogren's syndrome, celiac disease, intestinal parasites, Helicobacter pylori infection of the stomach, mold exposure, and lupus. At the end of the massive testing, Sammy was labeled as an "anxious patient." After four months, we had no answers. Just strange, apparently unrelated symptoms.

I was a tangle of anxiety. Some days, I'd come home from the grocery store and Sam would be stretched out on the couch, pale and sick. He'd struggle to go to work. Some evenings, he'd feel better, locking himself in his room with online LSAT practice tests. The symptoms would flare up and down, up and down, with no discernible pattern.

"Let's go back to the University of Florida to see Dr. Weinstein," I suggested. After several parental nudges, Sam agreed to the Florida trip.

Dr. Weinstein did a "tune-up" on Sam, measuring blood sugar and lactic acid for two days. I stepped out for many of the conversations between Sammy and Dr. Weinstein; after all, my son was twenty-two. In between nurse visits and Dr. Weinstein, we'd go visit the young GSD patients on the floor. The parents' eyes would light up when they'd see the six-foot-two, curly-headed hulk walk into the room. Sam represented hope to them. In a similar way, Sam's face brightened when Dr. Nadia made her rounds, clipboard in hand and an ever-present smile on her face. She was the first GSD patient to finish medical school and take her boards. Very simply, Dr. Nadia epitomized the future to Sam. He could dare to think about law school and beyond. Sam's happiness grew even more after one particular conversation with Dr. Weinstein. "You will live to play with your grandchildren," our saint assured Sam. "However, to do this, you have to manage your GSD health rigorously."

As the next few weeks progressed, Sam adhered to an adjusted cornstarch schedule, measuring out Argo precisely to the gram. We watched our food for unapproved GSD items, and Sam drank only water. Yet, the tiredness, foggy headedness, and GI symptoms continued.

Something was wrong with Sammy.

***

It became very clear that Sammy wasn't going to Spain for his language immersion. In between LSAT practice tests, he began searching online for medical help. One afternoon, Sam wandered out of his room, tapping his computer screen at me.

"The FODMAP diet, Mom." Sam gestured to the screen. "It stands for 'fermentable, oligosaccharides, disaccharides, monosaccharides, and polyols'—all hard-to-digest sugars and fibers that pass through the small intestine without being properly broken down."[1]

"But why does that cause a problem?"

"It says here, Mom, that when these FODMAPs pass into the colon, they ferment and create gas. They also pull water into the gut, and thereby stretch the intestines. This causes bloating, pain, cramping, diarrhea, or constipation. Also, maybe bacterial overgrowth."[2]

Sam and I sat together, reading on. "The low-FODMAP diet is a three-phase nutritional intervention. It includes an elimination phase, reintroduction phase, and personalization phase."[3]

"I'm going to print out the list of potential 'danger' foods," Sam continued. "Corn, garlic, onions, spinach . . . Can you work with this? All this new stuff on top of the GSD 'danger' foods?"

We soon ate very differently as a family.

***

Over the next six weeks, junk food disappeared from our home, as did pork, spinach, ramen noodles, butter, and bacon—the list was vast. We ate "safe" foods: grilled steak with olive oil, salt, and pepper. Plain baked potatoes. Sautéed

1. "What Is the Low FODMAP Diet?," Epicured, accessed May 15, 2020, https://mmm.epicured.com/low-fodmap-diet.
2. "Low FODMAP Diet."
3. "Low FODMAP Diet."

fresh kale. Steamed eggplant. Rice, sometimes, even though it was technically a FODMAP food. It appeared that limiting FODMAP foods was merely a baseline for the dietary changes Sammy needed to feel better. Sammy later learned that all meats had to be cooked fresh and eaten or frozen immediately, as histamines would build up quickly and disrupt the GI system. During this period of clean eating, Sammy also actively searched for a physician specializing in extreme food sensitivity. He reasoned that there had to be a medical system that functioned similarly to the methodology of lawyers: in other words, payment by the hour—and concrete results. Sam was tired of physicians who pushed him out the door after his allotted fifteen minutes. During the search for help, Sammy began to research, finding an article in the *Wall Street Journal* about a service called "Patient Navigator." Essentially, it was a company that would employ a researcher for any unique medical condition. The researcher, an individual with a PhD in the biological sciences, would take the hiring patient's symptoms and investigate extensively, coming up with a short list of possible medical conditions within a few weeks. It was a phenomenal concept. Our family was desperate to put a name and a definition on Sam's ailment. *We knew our son—he wasn't making these symptoms up.* Sam *was* anxious, of course, as the doctor's charts indicated. However, he was anxious because he battled cramps, nausea, and dizziness for no apparent reason. He was anxious because he wanted to get on with life. He was anxious because his symptoms were indicative of neurological problems, autoimmune problems, or infectious disease problems. He was anxious because he was truly eating according to the low-FODMAP diet yet experiencing marginal results. Was he just sick, or really, permanently sick? Worse than GSD sick, at the mere age of twenty-two?

"Mom, the deposit for the Patient Navigator research is $500.00. That money goes toward the hourly research fee of

$50.00. After that, you have to pay an additional hourly rate. Can we try this? I don't know what else to do, and I want to feel good again. I want to take the LSAT and go on to law school. The way I feel now, I can't do much of anything. I'm scared I'll spend the rest of my life lying on your couch." Sam sat next to me, the pages of the *Wall Street Journal* scattered around him. He rubbed his eyes, hollowed out and dull. My vital college grad was incapacitated, sitting on my couch, thirty pounds heavier than when he graduated, and we didn't know why. His life was going south fast. Where had my perky, confident son gone? I felt as lost as that night many years ago when Sammy cried and cried as a baby—and I couldn't help him. And I didn't know why *then* either. I didn't know.

Martin got home from a church meeting that day, and I grabbed him fast with the information on Patient Navigator. "What do you think?" I patted Martin's arm impatiently. All my years of living with GSD ambiguity had trained me well. I was sick at heart again, afraid to hope for a solution for Sam's misery. Could I hope, only to be smacked down again?

"We'll make it work," Martin reassured me. "We're parents, aren't we? I'm making a bit these days."

Within a day, we had Patient Navigator on board. I didn't want to get my hopes up too much. Sammy and I had seen so many experts over the past few months. Each one had her own paradigm, but no one had answers other than: "I can't find anything wrong." "Anxious." "Let's wait a couple of months and retest." "I'm going to refer you to ____ [fill in the blank]." Sam began filling in detailed pages of his medical information and emailed it off to Patient Navigator.

Miracles do happen. Within three weeks, Sam received an email backed with pages of data from Dr. Willingran, one of the researchers. I was elbow-deep in laundry when Sam bounded in. I hadn't seen any "bounding" from Sam in months, only an overweight, sluggish guy.

"This makes sense! I've been reading about this online!"

"What does the report say?" I slammed the dryer shut and peeked at the letter.

"Mast cell activation syndrome. MCAS."

I had never heard of mast cell activation syndrome, but I had never heard of glycogen storage disease a few years ago, either. Sam certainly had a knack for getting rare diseases.

"Mom, listen here." Sam read quickly, his hands shaking.

> "MCAS occurs when the mast cells in your body release too much of the substances inside them at the wrong times. These mast cells are part of your immune system. They're found in your bone marrow and around the blood vessels in your body. When you're exposed to stress or danger, your mast cells respond by releasing substances called mediators. Mediators cause inflammation, which helps your body heal from an injury or infection. This same response happens during an allergic reaction. Your mast cells release mediators to remove the thing you're allergic to. For example, if you're allergic to pollen, your mast cells release a mediator called histamine, which makes you sneeze to get rid of the pollen. If you have MCAS, your mast cells release mediators too frequently and too often."[4]

I looked over Sam's shoulder at the printout with a strange mix of anticipation and dread. What if? What if this new "thing" were like cancer? What if it were worse than GSD? Was this even fair for Sam to have *two* chronic health conditions? *Strike*

---

4. Nancy Moyer, "Mast Cell Activation Syndrome," Healthline, last modified July 13, 2022, https://www.healthline.com/health/mast-cell-activation-syndrome.

two, I thought, mentally shaking my finger at God. I remember touching Sam's arm, the skin so soft. "Sammy, maybe you're on to something!"

"Mom, right here it says that 'too many mediators can cause symptoms in *almost every system* in your body. However, the most commonly affected areas include your skin, nervous system, heart, and GI tract. Depending on how many mediators are released, your symptoms can range from mild to life-threatening.'"[5] Sam's finger scanned down the document rapidly. I just knew he wanted, so wanted, to get a diagnosis. The medical unknown was growing seeds of fear in him. "Here. Look right here. Itching skin. Runny nose. Swelling of the tongue. Trouble breathing. Low blood pressure. Mom, remember that time when I almost passed out in the bathroom? GI stuff here. Cramping, diarrhea, nausea. Nervous system also, Mom. Headaches, dizziness, confusion, extreme tiredness. Oh, my God. These are a lot of the symptoms that have been hitting me. They're all over my body. No wonder each specialist couldn't figure out the whole picture. They just thought I was a nutcase."

Sam and I sat at the kitchen table, reading page after page from Dr. Willingran. "Let's look at some of the triggers," I suggested. "Maybe that plus the low-FODMAP diet will help you to feel better over time." We scanned down the literature. There it was—our list of triggers to consider:

- allergic-type triggers, such as insect bites or certain foods
- drug-induced triggers, such as antibiotics, ibuprofen, and opiate pain relievers
- stress-related triggers, such as anxiety, pain, rapid temperature changes, exercise, being overly tired, or an infection

---

5. Moyer, "Mast Cell Activation Syndrome."

- smells, such as perfume
- hormonal changes, such as those related to a woman's menstrual cycle[6]

Sam began the lengthy process of identifying his own lifestyle triggers. "You know, Mom, when I take a hot shower, I feel kind of sick afterward. Also, being out in the sun. And after exercise." Sam's computer was open, and he pecked away on a new spreadsheet. I glanced at the columns. "Sammy Hayles. Symptom. Possible Cause. Time of day. Date. Comments." Sam was on it.

"So, we can't really identify troubling foods, yet?" I continued to hover, hopeful with the new information.

"Nope. I have to eat super clean for the next six weeks. Then, I can add one potential trigger food back in at a time. See here. I'll add those foods in on the spreadsheet when it's time."

"Look down here, Sam. Ways to determine if you truly have MCAS."

- Symptoms affect at least two body systems and are recurrent, and there's no other condition causing them.
- Blood or urine tests performed during an episode show you have higher levels of markers for mediators than you do when you aren't having an episode.
- Medications that block the effects of the mast cell mediators or their release make your symptoms go away.[7]

Sam and I kept skimming the data for how to control MCAS. "Here it is." Sam pointed. "Thank God. Not just food

6. Moyer, "Mast Cell Activation Syndrome."
7. Moyer, "Mast Cell Activation Syndrome."

control. If I can find a knowledgeable doc, here's some stuff I could try."

- H1 or H2 antihistamines. These drugs block the effects of histamines, which are one of the main mediators released by mast cells.
- Mast cell stabilizers. These drugs prevent the release of mediators from mast cells.

"Wow. This is easier said than done, right?" I tapped my finger on item one. "Figuring out if no other condition is causing your headaches or your GI issues? Isn't that what we've been investigating the past six months?"

"Yeah. Let me type in down here what all systems I've had tested so far."

The list was *long.* Sam and I began Googling for doctors familiar with MCAS. Unfortunately, that list was *short.* Turned out, MCAS was just as rare as glycogen storage disease, if not more so.

33

Crawling Forward

In the midst of symptom tracking and eating cleanly, Sammy had finished his Princeton Review class and had taken multiple practice LSAT exams.

"It's showtime," Sam announced one day as I folded laundry. "Wish me luck!"

I gave Sam a motherly hug. "I'm so proud of you, no matter how the LSAT comes out. You've been working at it so hard, and I know you've felt crappy for months. Don't know how you do it—you're just an amazing guy." Sam's hands felt cold and clammy; I could feel the nervousness flowing from him.

Sam arrived home a few hours later, his eyes bloodshot. He had worked with LSAT officials ahead of time so that he could eat a snack and do his cornstarch during the testing break after section three. He just knew he couldn't make it through the entire testing. Mental energy actually lowered his blood sugar, much like physical exercise.

"Oh, my God," was all he said as he sat down at the kitchen bar after the test. After a brief lunch, Sam zonked out in his room, coming to three hours later.

***

About four weeks later, it came. The envelope. I was fairly tap dancing in the family room with anticipation.

Sam ripped the envelope open, breaking into a beautiful smile—something we hadn't seen for a while. "Oh, man," he breathed. "These scores will get me into quite a few schools. Well, not Harvard. And I'm a point shy of qualifying for Duke."

Martin rounded the corner with groceries just as I smarted off to Sam. "Well, you slacker! I *guess* we'll keep you." Martin, Sam, and I had the best family hug you've ever seen. I grabbed onto Sam, thinking of all the times he was in the hospital, or all the times he couldn't eat pizza at a birthday party, or . . . or. It had come. Good news!

Sam applied to several law schools, much as he had done for undergrad: a "stretch" or two, moderately hard, and several "easy" ones, with the idea of "easy" rather relative. In a few weeks, he heard back about two free rides and a couple of reduced tuitions. "The one I really want is Georgetown Law Center. I could make some great connections there—and the professors! They're amazing. I'm scared to even dream it, but some day, I'd love to work for the Department of Justice. Both Georgetown and the DOJ are big stretches, though." Dr. Rittler's presence from Sam's high school days was alive and well, nudging my son's brain. Sam knew he couldn't change the world, but maybe reverse an unfair ruling? Maybe stop an antitrust violation?

Sam got wait-listed at Georgetown. Somewhat hopeful, he and I combed through the admission data. "Look here." I pointed at the information. "Says you can appeal in writing and submit a supplemental essay. What do you think?"

"I have to try. I just have to try." Sam wandered off to his room. He had just cooked himself some scrambled eggs to see if he could tolerate them—turned out, nope. They moved to the "potentially evil" list. At this point, he hadn't found a specialist to advise him. Patients with MCAS can have bad reactions to a number of foods, and often there's no rhyme or reason to what they can handle. The only way to find out is by trying a bit of the food and waiting to see how the body reacts. So, with eggs, Sam felt nauseated and exhausted within five minutes. Later, however, I heard insistent typing. Sam had logged in his egg reaction and then began hammering away on his Georgetown essay. Within three days, he had appealed his wait-listed status.

Three weeks later, Sam got another letter from Georgetown. The response lay on the kitchen counter, hopeful yet ominous. Sam circled the envelope like a stray dog eyeing a fresh bone. Finally, he tore into it, while I held my breath. "Come on, God," I prayed, trying to make a bargain with the Almighty. "Just let Sam go for it. Give him a chance!"

Sam got to "go for it." His wait-listed status at Georgetown became a full admission.

***

For the third time in his life, Sam prepared to head to school.

One day, he came out of his room, smiling. "Guess who I'm going to live with at school? Karthik!" I had forgotten that Karthik was studying at George Washington School of Medicine. His years of Saturday morning studying had paid off. I was sure that his mom and dad were busy now, working on the daughter, Anupama. I smiled, thinking of little Anu, who would hang around my kitchen cabinets, mooching Oreo cookies. "Karthik has an apartment with another guy in the Foggy Bottom area of DC. I can take the metro over to the law school every day." *Perfect,* I thought. *Living with a friend during law school would be comforting. And a future doctor, no less. Could Karthik help Sam in any way?*

Late that summer, Sam registered for classes. He was assigned to "Section A" of the L1 year, so the first year's classes would include Civil Procedure, Constitutional Law, Criminal Justice, Legal Practice: Writing and Analysis, Property, Torts, and International Law. We had gotten a partial student loan for tuition; Martin and I felt strongly that Sam would feel plenty of skin in the game if he, too, were paying tuition. Plus, it was a lot of money going out the door for us as a family.

That summer should have been one of joy. After all, Sam was heading toward one of his dreams—law school. Instead, it was a summer of horrible uncertainty.

As the end of August loomed, Sam was as sick as ever, despite his careful diet. He had been to about twenty doctors during the past year, but still had no real answers. Dr. Willingran's research indicated MCAS, but what did you do with that kind of diagnosis? What if Sam got to Washington, DC—six hours from us—and became even more ill? How could he manage the rigors of law school? The decision for law school was on and off due to his health. On and off.

He decided to push forward into life. He just *had to.* On a muggy day in late August, the three of us loaded up the SUV with clothes, a new comforter, toiletries, and cornstarch. Lots of cornstarch and a big bag of empty plastic containers and lids. Fortunately, the small bedroom Sam would use had a desk, a bookcase, one lamp, and a bed. The kitchen had pots, pans, and dishes. All the rooms were amply furnished with mice and assorted bugs. Since the apartment was right next door to George Washington University Hospital, it shook with blaring sirens day and night. But being that close to a hospital and an ER was a good thing.

All that said, it was an easy move-in. As we helped Sammy unpack, I fussed with Sam's computer and pencil cup obsessively, true to my nature as a mother and worrier. I felt anxious, like the time we moved Sam into camp at Bryn Mawr ten years ago. This time, the stakes were even higher. Sam would be far away from us again, tackling a law school regimen that was brutal even for a "normal" student, much less one who was chugging cornstarch every three hours.

Back home, I prayed daily for Sam to make it through the craziness of law school. The kids at Georgetown were bright *and* go-getters. I remember many times Martin talking of his law school experience, stating, "It was terrible. It was the armpit of my life back then." Sammy would go through that same awful "armpit period," I was afraid. Only he wasn't a typical, healthy twenty-three-year-old. He was a sick kid tackling seventeen-hour days.

About a week into school, I got a call from him that fluctuated between panic and a rant. "Oh, my God, Mom. On the first day of my Civil Procedures class, Professor Halton had us get out a piece of blank paper and write an 'original writ.' We all just sat there and looked at each other. What the heck is an 'original writ'? After about four minutes of all one hundred of us sitting with blank looks and even blanker paper, the professor said, 'I want you to remember how you feel right now. You don't know the answer to the question. In fact, you'll never know answers to the questions your clients bring you. It's going to be this way your whole career. It is up to *you,* and *you* alone, to research and battle with the issues.' Mom, I felt so stupid. What have I gotten myself into? I don't know if I can do law school."

"Sounds like everyone in class was stumped. And you're in school with a bunch of bright kids."

"And then!"—I heard a long, shaky breath—"In Constitutional Law, well, thank God I had read the assignment and briefed the cases. Remember *The Paper Chase*? Our professor was like Charles Kingsford grilling James Hart. One kid in the second row hadn't read his cases and tried to fake an answer. The professor had this guy in knots and tears in three minutes. I'm just petrified I'll get called on."

"But *you,* Sam, will have read and analyzed your cases. I know you."

"Yeah, I'm working like sixteen, seventeen hours a day. But if I accidentally get any food in me that my body doesn't like, I feel like crap for hours. I'm trying to analyze these cases sometimes, and my head just hurts so bad. Or, I get Montezuma's revenge."

"Keep writing down your foods and your symptoms, Sam. You, more than any of the doctors, can figure this out, because *you know you.*" I motioned for Martin to come talk with Sam. "He's panicked about analyzing all the cases," I whispered. "The horrible workload."

In the next thirty minutes, I heard Martin talk Sam "off the ledge." In his beautiful, calm manner, Martin recounted the times he, too, had been panicked in law school. "You'll get faster and faster in combing through a case for pertinent details," he reassured Sam. "It will go twice as fast in about two weeks. Stay with it. You can do this! We are just so proud of you and how hard you are working. This is a steady marathon, not a sprint. A step at a time."

Off the figurative ledge, Sam gulped a dose of cornstarch, ate a few saltines, and dove into *Marbury v. Madison.* I resolved to research doctors throughout the US who worked extensively with MCAS patients. Merely watching trigger foods was not cutting it for Sam. He was sick yet attempting to study many hours a day.

Only later did I find out how horrific his year one of law

school was. On one of our mother-and-son trips to Target to buy new tennis shoes, out it came. The first year.

Sam would take the metro to school each morning with his heavy pack of law books, snacks, and cornstarch. After he'd exit the metro, he'd walk an additional six blocks to McDonough Hall for his first class. It would take him about forty minutes of class time to shake off the nausea and exhaustion from the walk to class. After a full day on campus, he'd get back to the apartment in Foggy Bottom, sick again from just the commute.

In the evenings, Sam would pore over his cases and could only study for forty minutes, lie down for fifteen—study forty, lie down again. It was the only way he could make it through school.

I remember several times during year one of law school. I'd get a call:

"Mom!"

Then silence on the line.

"Sammy? Sammy? Are you okay?"

Just a shaky breath on the other line. Silence. More silence.

"Yeah, I guess. I'm sitting on a bench outside Whole Foods over on Pierce Street. I can't breathe. I can't . . . I can't . . ."

"Okay, Sammy. Do you feel weird, like you have stuff rising from your gut up into your lungs?"

"Yeah. Oh, my God, what is it? Oh, my God."

"Sounds like what your dad used to get when he was in law school. A panic attack. Just stay with me on the line. Breathe. I'm here. I'm here . . . and I love you. Let's just talk and give this a few moments." We'd chat about Professor Hardy with the huge wart on his forehead, or *Palsgraf v. Long Island Railroad Company*, or about roommate Karthik's interesting diet of aloo gobi.

Soon, a regular breath. More minutes would pass.

"Sam, are you okay now?"

"I think so."

A breath. One more.

Eventually, Sammy would rally and head back to his apartment.

"I'm good now, Mom. Thanks. Love you!"

"Me, too, Buster. I love you thiiiiiiiiiiis much!"

I'd hang up, and my heart would break. Just break.

***

Back in North Carolina, I sighed after a particularly heartrending conversation with Sam. I researched and Googled, trying to find a specialist familiar with MCAS. Just as GSD had been twenty years earlier, MCAS was an unknown. For years, patients lived with this terrible disorder, yet often became horribly dysfunctional over time or died from anaphylactic shock. Some patients had to go on full disability, unable to even leave their homes. Additionally, because they complained of multisystem ailments to their physicians, many became labeled as "whiners and anxious." Management of the condition eventually fell into two realms: H1 or H2 antihistamines that could block the effects of histamines, a type of mediator released by mast cells. Or, some medications, called mast cell stabilizers, could prevent the release of mediators from mast cells in the first place. Sam was attempting to prevent the release of mediators by eating correctly. It was not enough. The next day, I wailed about this situation to my internist during my annual checkup. Dr. Powell had probed a bit when she saw my blood pressure. "What's going on in your life?" She looked concerned, listening as though she had all day. Quietly, she wrote down five important words for me on a Post-it note: "Lawrence Afrin, MD: MCAS specialist."

I called Sam that night amidst his pile of casework, telling him about the expert in MCAS. "Dr. Afrin practices out of Armonk, New York. Maybe after your December break, we can both fly to White Plains for an initial consult." I agreed to do some legwork to get an appointment set up.

I worked hard during October to get a January appointment with Dr. Afrin. Sam was not a minor, so that was roadblock one—I couldn't make the appointment for him. Also, he was in DC, knee-deep in study outlines and a study group when he wasn't in class. Dr. Afrin was in New York and tied up with countless patients. I felt like I couldn't talk to anyone. As it turned out, too, Sam had to "prove" that he had one of the indicators of MCAS. Just feeling horrible most of the time was not enough.

"Remember about a year ago when you had a colonoscopy and an endoscopy? It was when we were trying to figure out what was wrong with you. Well, Dr. Afrin will accept data from your biopsies. Apparently, the cell blocks from the biopsies can be stained, so mast cells can be detected. Anyway, Sam, can you make some calls and get this sent to him? I can't do this because of HIPAA, of course." The patient privacy laws were strict.

Sam got the data sent. Would Dr. Afrin accept Sam as a case study?

34

Medication and More Medication

The wind whipped around the White Plains airport, rattling the windows with icy blasts. I had lived in what we called "North Cackalacky" for five years and had acclimated; I'd grab a parka and earmuffs when the temperature dropped to fifty. That day in White Plains, it was a bracing fourteen degrees. As I sat in the terminal waiting area, I felt excited to meet up with Sam and perhaps get help. He had made it through his first semester of law school, declaring that the final exams were brutal. He had slept for two days off and on after he finished, then took the train to Chapel Hill for three days of Christmas break. He had gone back to DC early to buy textbooks and begin reading for the second semester classes. By January, Sam had no clue if he had passed his classes. With one midterm and one final per class, it was a make-or-break situation. Sure, you could get an A, B, or a C in each class, but those Cs wouldn't get you much of a career later on.

Our time with Dr. Afrin was helpful, despite the chilling blasts that shook my southern soul. How had I turned into a warm-weather wimp in five years?

He had reviewed the colonoscopy biopsies and ordered massive blood work as well as a twenty-four-hour urine collection. Laboratory tests for evidence of MCAS included things I had never heard of: serum chromogranin A, histamine and prostaglandin, N-methylhistamine, dinor 11-beta-PGF2-apha, and leukotriene E4.[1] The specialist also told Sam that MCAS could reveal itself in many random symptoms, including throat pain, prostatitis, chronic pelvic pain, nonbacterial cystitis, general sensitivity to pain, diarrhea, nausea, asthma, cognitive fogginess, or anxiety. After three days, Sam flew back to DC, hopeful and waiting on test results. "There are a lot of alternatives we can try," Dr. Afrin had reassured Sam. "It's different with each person, and you have to work in one medication at a time, just like you would a new food. Otherwise, you don't know what is actually helping you. It's trial and error for each person." In other words, MCAS had no quick fix, just management.

The second year of law school. Hope. Sam had gotten several As and a few Bs during year one. He had been so sick that year, struggling just to get to class and back. However, it wasn't until Sam's second year of law school that he began medications to truly manage MCAS. While he continued FaceTime calls with Dr. Afrin, he also discovered an allergist only a block away from his apartment, very close to the George Washington University Hospital. The young woman had worked with several MCAS patients. Most importantly, this specialist was one of the first physicians to acknowledge Sam's personal knowledge of his conditions. Between the two specialists, Sam began

1. "Mast Cell Activation Syndrome (MCAS)," American Academy of Allergy, Asthma, and Immunology, accessed May 15, 2020, https://www.aaaai.org/Conditions-Treatments/related-conditions/mcas.

to painstakingly test several medications, one by one, while also monitoring his FODMAP diet.

Both of Sam's new doctors recommended that he start on a combination of H1 and H2 blockers—to "wall off" mast cell mediators. Because Sam experienced system-wide symptoms, he would be taking both H1 and H2 blockers.

For H1 blockers, patients often take Zyrtec (cetirizine), Claritin (loratadine), or Allegra (fexofenadine). Common H2 blockers include Zantac (ranitidine), Pepcid AC (famotidine), Tagamet (cimetidine), or Axid (nizatidine). At the present time, the FDA has banned ranitidine and its brand name Zantac for possible carcinogenic ingredients. On the other hand, to stabilize mast cells, specialists often recommend oral cromolyn or ketotifen, mixed with water about four times daily before meals. Many times, patients must take both medications, which are available at compounding pharmacies.

Other recommendations exist for the condition. MCAS patients must avoid certain drugs that trigger mast cell release, including narcotics, muscle relaxants, certain antibiotics, antiseizure drugs, local anesthetics, IV dye, and ACE inhibitors.[2] To promote overall health, MCAS patients may often take probiotic therapies.

Does this all sound like a lot of medications and diet manipulation? You bet.

At Dr. Afrin's instruction, Sam began taking thirty milligrams of levocetirizine daily. This over-the-counter medication, commonly known as Xyzal, was an antihistamine working to block the young man's reactions to hot showers, perfume, certain lotions and shampoos, and bright sunlight. The second prescription Sam began was two milligrams of oral ketotifen daily. This drug is often used for the treatment of

2. Daniel Elieh Ali Komi and Leif Bjermer, "Mast Cell-Mediated Orchestration of the Immune Responses in Human Allergic Asthma: Current Insights," *Clinical Reviews in Allergy & Immunology* 56 (April 2019); 234–247, https://doi.org/10.1007/s12016-018-8720-1.

asthma, food allergies, anaphylaxis, irritable bowel syndrome, and general MCAS issues.

Just imagine. Each day, Sam had to think about which soap, which shampoo to use in the morning, also making sure his shower was lukewarm—not hot. He had to think about every morsel of food that went into his mouth all day long. He had to manage doses of cornstarch every three hours as well as oral ketotifen four times daily. If he went to a seminar or meeting at school, he had to bypass all pizza—all beer. On the commute to and from classes, Sam had to wear sunglasses and a hat to keep the sun from starting a migraine. If he had to break into a fast walk to get to class, he felt sick. His life was hemmed in on all sides.

I knew what Sam could eat because I had cooked for him during his summer breaks. I can tell you; it wasn't much. And the trigger foods at first glance appeared random. For example, Sam would react to peanuts, but not Brazil nuts. Salt and pepper were okay, but not rosemary or chives. He could eat sautéed kale, but not spinach. Fresh sea bass was okay, but not salmon. The other huge difficulty: rice could be "in" one week and "out" the next. The target moved, continually.

***

After Sam's visit with Dr. Afrin and his local allergist, he continued testing various foods for reactions and worked in one medication at a time, according to his physicians' advice. Sundays became Sam's day to buy groceries for the week. He'd walk everything back to his apartment and begin cooking—a two-hour production. All food would be frozen immediately in small ziplock bags. The apartment freezer was bulging with baggies of cooked ground turkey (absent rosemary seasoning). Other baggies contained icy chunks of steamed kale, cooked eggplant, or new potatoes. The cabinets were full of potato chips cooked in coconut oil, Brazil nuts, dried kelp, cornstarch, plastic cornstarch containers, Citrucel, and probiotics. It looked like a science lab. During the busy week, Sam would microwave a bit of food for breakfast and then pack lunch into a thermal pouch filled with four ice blocks. The lunch, along with the day's measured cornstarch and medication, all fit into Sam's backpack, along with three or four law books and spiral notebooks. During the thirty-minute commute to Georgetown Law, he lugged the heavy pack.

Sam's second semester of year two went better. Sometimes he'd have several days at a time when he felt good. Occasionally, if he tried a new probiotic, he would experience two days of nausea and exhaustion. Unfortunately, the crush of law school study never stopped—not for Saturdays and Sundays, not for GSD, and not for MCAS. I'm not sure where it was that Sam reached for strength and determination to keep studying. He had only what I can describe as "grit," a relentless, laser-focused desire to finish law school and to do so cum laude.

After writing about fifty application letters, Sam obtained a summer unpaid internship with Judge Ann Marie Calabria with the North Carolina Court of Appeals in Raleigh. He planned to live with us and drive my car, since his old clunker had been sold when he went off to law school. There were few parking spots in DC; besides, we needed the money to pay for all the law books. I volunteered to cook for him that summer, because with the hour commute twice daily, he'd be gone ten hours a day.

It was during this internship in 2018 that Sam experienced the feeling of actually practicing law. He researched cases for Judge Calabria eight hours a day and loved it. Our standard family joke ran like this:

Mom: "So, what case are you working on now? Anything interesting?"

Sam: "I'm loving the research! Well, I can't tell you about the case."

Mom (with Joisey accent and hands on hips): "Seriously? You talkin' to me? Come on—just tell me a little. I'm your mudder, for Pete's sake."

Sam: "Nope."

Mom: "But—"

Sam: "Nope."

And on it went.

At this point in Sam's life, he had the management of his GSD and MCAS fairly well worked out. That summer, you should have seen our kitchen. We had a clean towel on the counter with a large covered bowl of cornstarch and six clean plastic containers, resting upside down. We had a gram scale out. Sam's string pack lay nearby. Levocetirizine, ketotifen, ranitidine, and vials of cromolyn were lined up on the counter. Inside the pantry were piles of new potatoes, blocks of dried kelp, boxes of Argo cornstarch, baggies of Brazil nuts, and Jackson's Honest Chips. Our freezer was packed with pouches of cooked turkey, eggplant, and kale.

Working for Judge Calabria was definitely *not* 'Sup Dog. Sam had to wear a dress shirt each day. A backpack just didn't quite look right in this new job. But what to do? Even before the internship started, Sam obsessed about appearing "normal" in the workaday world. What would the other clerks think when he had to microwave his frozen crumbled turkey and eggplant or shake up mysterious white powder in water? What if he was having a bad MCAS day and had to run to the restroom six times? How would he transport his frozen lunch and cornstarch bottles to work each day discreetly? Sam had told his direct supervisor at work that he had "GI problems," but not Judge Calabria. GI problems. That was an understatement, as Sam juggled two chronic conditions.

"What if there's a special end-of-summer lunch for us interns? What if people want to go out after work to a bar? What am I going to do?" Somehow, Sam had gotten through most of childhood with only moderate anxiety about his conditions. However, he was stressing now. I think that he really wanted to make a go of a career. Would being ill impact his hiring chances? Would he be perceived as weak, unable to do his job?

***

We got on Amazon and searched for leather satchels. That one, there—the dignified oxblood leather one. It would look better than the beaten-up backpack from law school. Hmmmm. Could Sam cram in his refrigerated lunch carrier, plastic blocks of ice, four cornstarch containers, a water bottle, and his computer?

Guess what. The leather satchel worked. Sam looked "normal," like every other intern in Judge Calabria's service. Except he wasn't, of course.

The summer blew by, and in late August, Sam was back in DC for his third and final year of law school. It went well, for a while. Sam had decided to restart the defunct antitrust club at school, recruiting new members and hosting informational seminars for fellow students. Various law professors were normally good about presenting at the seminars. The antitrust club would have free pizza afterward, with Sam nervously working the crowd, Brazil nuts in hand.

Mid-fall 2018, Sam began complaining to me about various foods that set off nausea and exhaustion. Chicken and rice, former staples, suddenly became off-limits. Why? Then, corn really began to bother Sam. That normally would not have been a deal breaker, but Argo cornstarch—the lifeblood of a patient with GSD—was corn. It was a high-stakes problem. Cornstarch and food literally kept Sam alive. Without them, Sam's blood sugar would plummet to thirty within a few hours. He'd be dead in less than twenty-four hours or hooked up to an IV in a hospital. *Really?* I questioned God. *You let Sam get to law school, have him do well, and now this? Really?* My spirituality wavered. I was angry and just plain worn-out after twenty-three years of Sam's health struggles.

That semester, I could feel Sam's anxiety simply vibrating whenever he'd call. The year he'd lived with us, his weight had increased to 245 pounds—a bit heavy, even for a six-foot-two fellow. With the new food allergies emerging, Sam could eat less and less. Soon, he dropped to *ten* foods and weighed only 185 pounds. When he'd do his cornstarch dose—every three hours—he'd feel nauseated for two hours afterward. Then he'd rally for an hour, only to take another cornstarch dose and fight the nausea again. There seemed no way out of this. Sam had to take his cornstarch to keep his blood sugar up. On top of this, Sam was studying like a fiend. He wanted to get all As his 3L year, to boost his GPA enough to make cum laude. The situation was absolute misery personified as Sam dragged through each day. Would he shrink to eating four foods? Unknown. What if he couldn't handle cornstarch? Bad news. The worst of news.

I began digging into research again, trying to keep Sam relatively free to begin his outlines for the December final exams. I turned desperately to Dr. Weinstein for help, setting up a conference call between the specialist and Sam.

"Honestly, I've never had a GSD patient who suffers from mast cell issues," Dr. Weinstein had told Sam on the call.

"Did you get any guidance at all?" I had asked Sam that afternoon. *What were we going to do without Argo?* I picked at a cuticle anxiously, making myself bleed. *Here we are again, in totally uncharted territory. How long, God, are we going to do this?*

"Well, Dr. Weinstein did say I could try Authentic Foods Tapioca Flour instead of cornstarch. Apparently, it will keep my blood sugar up as well as Argo. He said there are other flours, too, like almond, amaranth, barley, chickpea, and rice flours. They don't work as well for sugar control. So I guess I'll begin working in tapioca flour gradually tomorrow. See what happens. Mom, what if it doesn't work?"

Yes, *what if it doesn't work?* It would be a death sentence.

My mind couldn't go to the "what if." "Sounds like a plan," I reassured Sam. A bit of tension seeped out of me. "I'll dig around on the MCAS website—see what I can find about food problems. Other people *must* be going through these same issues."

"Yeah, and some of those people are incapacitated. They can't even leave their apartments. They can't work."

"Hang on. Just hang on. Let me research. Hey, I love you thiiiiiiiiis much!" I started digging into information fast, my gut churning with anxiety—an all-too-familiar churn.

***

Sammy actually spent two hours of poking around the MCAS website, somehow packing this search into the incredible workload. He found a name. A name and a solution, perhaps?

Lucinda Williams was a registered dietitian who worked solely with mast cell patients. She used tried-and-true techniques to help her patients work problem foods back in. That was what Sam needed desperately. He set up a conference call with Ms. Williams the following week.

"You won't believe this, Mom." I could hear beeping in the background. Apparently, Sam was microwaving dinner—turkey, new potatoes, and kale. "So, it's a rotational thing. The first two weeks, I pick out a food I really want to work back into my diet. I think I might start with chicken. So, I'll eat like one little sliver of cooked chicken on Monday. Wait a day. On Wednesday, two little slivers. You keep on like that, increasing just a bit on alternate days, until you can tolerate a full serving. Ms. Williams says that at first, I might feel a bit sick when I test. Well, then I work in the next food. I'm gonna try rice, then green beans."

I was amazed. My very own grandfather had eaten a rotational diet in the early 1900s. I never knew much about the venerable attorney who lived in Pittsburg, Kansas, other than he had asthma and food allergies. Huh. Maybe I had passed down the mast cell problem along with GSD.

Sam was able to work in chicken, rice, and green salads over the next few months. But not green beans. With only one measly bean, he felt sick in minutes. But, over time, food introduction worked. Sam went from eating only ten foods to twenty. It was a miracle. It was a testament to eating carefully, tracking foods, and personal discipline, week after week.

***

The end of Sam's final year of law school was a blur of cases, outlines, study groups, and grueling final exams. It was a blur of tapioca starch, FODMAP rules, levocetirizine, and ketotifen.

In mid-May 2019 Thomas, Martin, and I arrived in Washington. It was *hot* that day. It was a Washington, DC, *sticky* hot. It didn't matter. Sam was graduating from law school.

We sat in makeshift wooden camp chairs, surrounded by four hundred other parents, grandparents, and assorted screaming children. The wooden slats of the chairs pleated our hindquarters as sweat trickled down our backs and in front of our ears.

I fanned myself with the Georgetown Law program and perched on the edge of my chair, hoping to see the students better. It was a sea of twentysomethings out there, all dressed in heavy black robes and eight-sided tams. Each graduate sported a purple cord on the tam and a heavy purple stole lying over the black robe.

Two o'clock approached. We could all feel expectation build and crest, as grandparents and parents fanned and waited, fanned and waited. I looked for my son. Not that row—maybe the next? No. Hayles. Maybe in the middle.

I scanned the young law school students as they chatted with each other in anticipation. And then—I found my son. His eyes spotted mine across the sea of black and purple. Blazing blue eyes behind navy glasses. Dark curls flipping over the tam. Standing tall above the others, he flashed us a huge grin and a thumbs-up.

A single chime echoed across Healy Lawn from the bell tower on campus. The students and law professors stood in a sudden whoosh, while cadets marched the US and Georgetown flags to the back of the stage, slowly, sedately, to Pachelbel's Canon in D. I heard name after name. Student after student. My skin started to prickle in excitement. And then—*Sammy Hayles: juris doctor, cum laude.*

I grabbed Martin's hand and then Tee's. *Thank you, God. Just—thank you.*

***

Today, Sam works for a corporate law firm based in DC. He handles litigation upon occasion, but also works on multibillion-dollar mergers. Attorneys on the team must ensure that the buyout doesn't create antitrust issues. In his spare time, which is minimal, he plays the drums, hangs with friends, and watches improv. And—I hear something about a lady named Samantha.

35

The So What of It All

It seems easy to look back on the past twenty-nine years and pontificate. Yes, we did this and investigated that. We researched this and tried that. The reality is the Hayles family bumbled through Sam's medical conditions quite a bit. However, amidst the confusion and mapless journey, we did manage to learn. Sammy has grown up to be a fully functioning adult in a career he loves. So, what's the "so what" of my learnings?

- When you learn you have a child with a chronic disability or illness, make a comprehensive list of everyone you know who could help you—either emotionally or practically.
- Relish any and all improvements you see in your child. It may be finally getting that smile from him or seeing him eat on his own.

- Share setbacks and frustrations with trusted family members or friends.
- Research, research, research! Physicians and specialists are wonderful, but you know your child the best. You are also the person who will push the hardest for him. Specialists tend to have a particular viewpoint or paradigm—they are, after all, human. You will need to cross paradigms all the time.
- Teach your child about his condition by involving him in his daily care.
- As best as you can, have your child assume family responsibilities.
- Don't assume your child can't perform a task. He'll often surprise you.
- Set small achievable goals of independence for your child. Look for new opportunities for him to "stretch." Baby steps can become adult steps, but it may take months or years.
- Document your child's condition, ER instructions, and medical schedule. Have a power of attorney ready to use when you travel to a new city or country.
- Make sure all medical supplies are available. Redundancy is always good.
- Ask for help and be kind to yourself. Check with trusted friends or relatives so you can have a day off. Perhaps take your other children out for a treat. You're in a long marathon, not a sprint.
- Celebrate *how hard* your child is working, not just the actual end event.
- *Listen* to your child. What is he feeling and fearing? Talk with him.
- Join a group of others who have the same

condition. Share knowledge, pain, and frustration. It feels good to know you're not out there alone. Try to . . .

Whoops. I have to go. Sammy's on the phone. My old enemies, fear and anxiety, grab me by the hand and lead me down my twenty-nine-year path of fear. What's wrong? Is it Sam's GSD? Is it his mast cell? *Oh dear oh dear oh dear oh dear.*

No, it's a "happy call," with news about Sam's great job review and lady love, Samantha. Sometimes, life is just darn *good.*

APPENDIX

The Walk to Hope

For the first time in history, we parents, caregivers, and patients with GSD 1a have hope! Humans can potentially have their GSD 1a "fixed." In 1971, the year of my high school graduation, the disease was almost always fatal. And now—fifty years later—there's a chance. A chance.

While research in MCAS is still in its infancy, glycogen storage disease type 1 has been a recognized and defined condition since 1929. Strides toward managing the condition evolved in the early 1970s with the discovery of Argo cornstarch as a blood-sugar management tool. Additionally, while Sammy had to be definitively diagnosed with GSD 1a via two liver biopsies in 1993, the process is easier today. According to Rarediseases.org,

> GSD type I is diagnosed by laboratory tests that indicate abnormal levels of glucose, lactate, uric acid, triglycerides and cholesterol . . . or a liver biopsy. . . .[1]

1. "Glycogen Storage Disease Type I," Rare Disease Database, NORD, accessed May 20, 2020, https://rarediseases.org/rare-diseases/glycogen-storage-disease-type-i/.

What is on the research horizon today for GSD 1a? In a word, gene therapy. Ultragenyx Pharmaceuticals has developed a therapy called DTX401—an "investigational AAV gene therapy being developed for the potential treatment for patients with glycogen storage disease type 1a. DTX401 is designed to address the defective gene for the enzyme glucose-6-phosphatase-α, a defect that results in the inability to regulate blood sugar (glucose)."[2] In simpler English, this means that "an injection to the bloodstream delivers a normal copy of the defective gene to the liver, using a virus."[3] In essence, the dysfunctional gene becomes replaced.

The path to the Ultragenyx gene therapy for humans has been slow and meticulous. As the website CureGSD describes, in 2007, the University of Florida research team began working with Maltese dogs, the only canine species in which GSD occurs naturally. Maltese dogs affected by GSD 1a normally die within hours of their birth; even with cornstarch, the dogs typically die within four weeks. In 2007, Dulce, a Maltese with GSD 1a, received the first experimental gene therapy. CureGSD reports that

> within 2 weeks, the duration of fasting markedly increased, and visually the dog improved with decreased hepatomegaly, increased energy, and improved growth. The effect of gene therapy waned, so a second gene therapy was performed in January 2008. Following this treatment on Dulce, the lactate concentration normalized, and she was able to fast for 9

---

2. "DTX401: AAV8 Gene Therapy for Glycogen Storage Disease Type Ia (GSDIa)," Ultragenyx, accessed May 20, 2020, https://www.ultragenyx.com/pipeline/dtx-401-for-gsd1a/.
3. Carmen Leitch, "Remarkable Results from First Gene Therapy for Glycogen Storage Disease," Labroots, September 20, 2019, https://www.labroots.com/trending/genetics-and-genomics/15701/remarkable-results-gene-therapy-glycogen-storage-disease.

hours without development of hypoglycemia. All glucose support was stopped at 6 months of age, and Dulce had no problems clinically while weaning off therapy.[4]

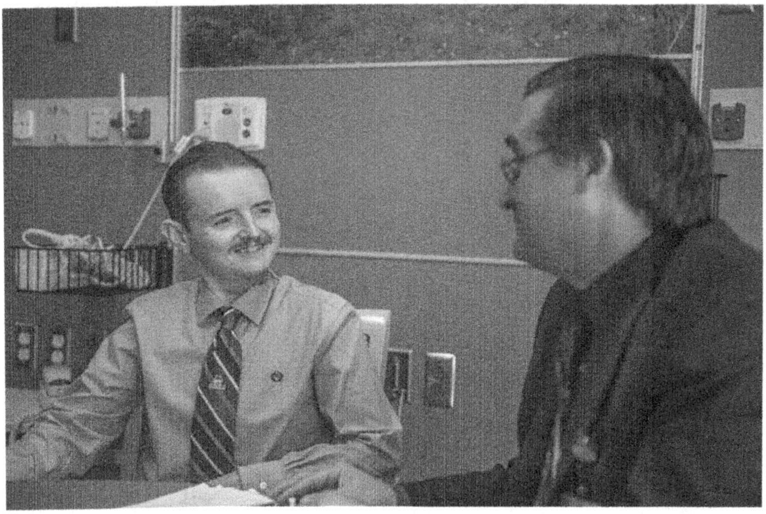

Jerrod Watts, a patient enrolled in the first clinical trial for glycogen storage disease, chatting with lead investigator Dr. David Weinstein

Researchers performed a liver biopsy on Dulce after the second gene therapy and determined that her liver was demonstrating 7 percent activity in converting glycogen to glucose. The website reports that twenty-one months after the second gene treatment, Dulce went into heat and, as a result, developed increased lactic acid. Dulce then went onto low-dose glucose therapy; she received her third gene therapy in 2010. Researchers report that at four years of age, Dulce has no "adenomas or evidence of complications."[5]

4. "Gene Therapy," CureGSD, accessed October 9, 2018, now available at "Gene Therapy," University of Florida Health, https://ufhealth.org/diabetes-center-excellence/research.
5. "Gene Therapy," CureGSD.

Dulce later gave birth to Tucker and Jasmine in 2010, with each puppy receiving gene therapy "using a modified vector."[6] At two weeks of age, both Tucker and Jasmine could fast for six hours; glucose support was discontinued at three weeks. A second gene-therapy treatment was performed when each pup was eight weeks of age. At the time of the website writing, both were doing well.

***

When I talked with Dr. Weinstein nearly eight years ago, I was amazed that the gene-therapy dosing would move directly from Maltese dogs to humans.

In typical pharmaceutical drug testing, animals are dosed with a new drug, with higher and higher levels of the drug administered. Then, human testing (clinical trials) incorporates a four-phase process.

In typical human FDA testing, Phase One represents a small group of young, healthy males that receives dosing of a new drug. Phase Two consists of a small group of individuals who have the targeted disease. Phase Three of the study involves hundreds or thousands of people with the disease. And finally, Phase Four occurs after FDA approval of the new drug. In this phase, the drug is tested for other applications.

After months and months of searching, Dr. Weinstein and fellow researchers entered into an agreement with Ultragenyx, a biopharmaceutical company focused on the development of novel products for rare and ultra-rare diseases. The company announced that on July 26, 2018, the first human patient was dosed "in the Phase 1/2 study of DTX401, an adeno-associated virus vector based on gene therapy for the treatment of patients with GSD 1a."[7] Ultragenyx states that the DTX401 "has

---

6. "Gene Therapy," CureGSD.
7. "Ultragenyx Announces First Patient Dosed in Phase 1/2 study of DTX401,

been shown in preclinical studies to improve G6Pase-a activity and reduce hepatic glycogen levels, a well-described biomarker of disease progression."[8] Also important is that the FDA has granted a Fast Track designation to DTX401 for the treatment of GSD 1a. According to Globenewswire, "The FDA Fast Track program is designed to facilitate the development and expedite the review of drugs that are intended to treat serious conditions and fill an unmet medical need. Fast Track designation allows for more-frequent interaction with the FDA review team."[9]

Ultragenyx described the Phase 1/2 GSD gene-therapy study as "open-label, dose-finding." The company also outlined several success factors of the study, including time to hypoglycemia, impact on lipids, uric acid levels, and measurement of glycogen in the liver. The company stated the testing protocol: "There are three potential dosing cohorts in the study, and three patients will be enrolled in each cohort. Patients in the first cohort receive a single dose of DTX401 of 2.0 x 10^12 GC/kg. The decision to proceed to the next, higher-dose cohort will be made after the data-monitoring committee evaluates the safety data for all patients in the previous dosing cohort."[10]

The human impact of the gene-therapy study has been huge. In 2019, Dr. Weinstein spoke at the Association for Glycogen Storage Disease's Forty-First Annual Conference,

---

a Gene Therapy for the Treatment of Glycogen Storage Disease Type Ia (GSDIa); FDA Grants Fast Track Designation to Gene Therapy Program," Ultragenyx, July 26, 2018, https://www.globenewswire.com/news-release/2018/07/26/1542689/0/en/Ultragenyx-Announces-First-Patient-Dosed-in-Phase-1-2-study-of-DTX401-a-Gene-Therapy-for-the-Treatment-of-Glycogen-Storage-Disease-Type-Ia-GSDIa-FDA-Grants-Fast-Track-Designation-t.html.

8. "Ultragenyx Announces First Patient Dosed."
9. "Ultragenyx Announces First Patient Dosed."
10. Lauren Woods, "World's Top Researcher of Rare Genetic Liver Disease Coming to Conn Health," *UConn Today*, September 19, 2016, https://today.uconn.edu/2016/09/worlds-top-glycogen-storage-disease-program-coming-uconn-health/.

describing the one-year clinical trial results with gene therapy as "remarkable."[11] Jerrod Watts, the first GSD patient to be treated, would agree. Following his gene therapy with wakeful IV infusion, Jerrod no longer requires up to a pound of cornstarch per day to regulate his glucose levels. Additionally, he has more energy and has been able to lose weight, as the high levels of cornstarch he needed to survive represented over 1,700 calories per day. Remarkably, these life-saving benefits have resulted from a gene-therapy dose only one-third of the required dose strength. "I can now sleep through the night without worrying about dying in the middle of the night. . . . I'm living, breathing proof that there is a light at the end of the tunnel with GSD."[12] Jerrod's message for other patients: "Please don't give up hope."[13]

As of first quarter 2022, Ultragenyx has completed its third cohort for gene therapy, a blinded control trial.[14] (J. Walker, "Ground-Breaking Clinical Trial Participant First in the World to Receive Phase III Infusion for GSD Type 1a," UConn Health, January 20, 2022). Although Dr. Weinstein has passed the GSD research torch to pursue studies in other rare disorders, the study continues, led by Dr. Rebecca Riba-Wolman at Connecticut Children's/UConn Health.

Each third cohort patient will receive an approximate forty-five-minute IV of the investigational product to test its safety and dosage levels.[15] Dr. Riba-Wolman explains that the gene therapy carries a "naturally occurring virus to the liver to replace deficient sugar enzymes caused by the disease and

---

11. Leitch, "Remarkable Results."
12. Leitch, "Remarkable Results."
13. Leitch, "Remarkable Results."
14. Jennifer Walker, "Ground-Breaking Clinical Trial Participant First in the World to Receive Phase III Infusion for GSD Type 1a," *UConn Today*, January 20, 2022, https://today.uconn.edu/2022/01/ground-breaking-clinical-trial-participant-first-in-the-world-to-receive-phase-iii-gene-therapy-for-gsd-type-ia/.
15. Walker, "Ground-Breaking Clinical Trial."

to jumpstart the body's glucose control."[16] After three days of an inpatient stay in the clinical trial unit for monitoring, the patient will wear a Dexcom continuous glucose monitor to provide follow-up information to the GSD study coordinators. Every three months, the participant will return to UConn Health for a fasting study.[17]

The study will take two years, but "after the first year, anyone receiving the placebo will be switched over to the investigational product."[18] The results and findings of Phase Three of the trial will be published and peer-reviewed, with the eventual goal of treatment for all those who have GSD 1a.

***

Imagine the excitement: people with GSD have a chance. We see exciting steps forward . . . to the walk to independence. Perhaps "every three hours" will just become a bad memory to many.

16. Walker, "Ground-Breaking Clinical Trial."
17. Walker, "Ground-Breaking Clinical Trial."
18. Walker, "Ground-Breaking Clinical Trial."

REFERENCES

American Academy of Allergy, Asthma, and Immunology. "Mast Cell Activation Syndrome (MCAS)." American Academy of Allergy, Asthma, and Immunology. Accessed May 15, 2020. https://www.aaaai.org/Conditions-Treatments/related-conditions/mcas.

Annabi, Borhane, Hisayuki Hiraiwa, Brian C. Mansfield, Ke-Jian Lei, Tsuneyuki Ubagai, Mihael H. Polymeropoulos, Shimon W. Moses, et al."The Gene for GSD Type 1b Maps to Chromosome 11q23," AJHG 62, no. 2 (February 1998). Accessed March 13, 2020. https://doi.org/10.1086/301727.

Beach, Randall S. *Shadow Child.* USA: Outskirts Press, 2017.

Busick, J. A. *Cora Means Heart: Memoirs of a Special Needs Mom.* (CreateSpace Independent Publishing Platform, 2018.

Chen, Margaret A., and David A. Weinstein. "Glycogen Storage Diseases: Diagnosis, Treatment and Outcome." *Translational Science of Rare Diseases* 1, no. 1 (August 2016): 45–72.

Chhabra, Sapna. "India Harbors Superbugs Everywhere—Do We Care?" *Research Matters.* April 13, 2018. Accessed April 27, 2020. https://researchmatters.in/news/india-harbors-superbugs-everywhere-%E2%80%93-do-we-care.

Crane, Kristine. "UF Pediatrician Earns Global Recognition for Treating Rare Disease." *Gainesville Sun* January 9, 2013.

https://www.gainesville.com/story/news/2013/01/09/uf-pediatrician-earns-global-recognition-for-treating-rare-disease/31841484007/.

Crisp, Claire. *Waking Mathilda*. USA: Palace Gates Press, 2017.

CureGSD. "Gene Therapy." Accessed October 9, 2018 (page discontinued).

Dempsey, Sharon. *Extreme Parenting*. Great Britain: Athenaeum Press, 2008.

"Disability." Google search. Accessed February 5, 2020. https://www.google.com/search?rlz=1C5CHFA_enUS778US778&ei=NXk8XoC9K6eltgXg4rWgCg&q=definition+of+a+disability&oq.

Epicured. "What Is the Low FODMAP Diet?" Accessed May 15, 2020. https://mmm.epicured.com/low-fodmap-diet.

Gardiner, Juliet. "The Story of Women in the 1950s." *History Today* 65, no. 9 (September 2015). Accessed February 27, 2020. https://www.historytoday.com/reviews/story-women-1950s.

Komi, Daniel Elieh Ali., and Leith Bjermer. "Mast Cell-Mediated Orchestration of the Immune Responses in Human Allergic Asthma: Current Insights." *Clinical Reviews in Allergy & Immunology* 56 (April 2019): 234–247. Accessed August 12, 2022. https://doi.org/10.1007/s12016-018-8720-1.

Larsen, Pamala D. *Lubkin's Chronic Illness*. Boston, MA: Jones and Bartlett Learning, 2019.

Learning RX. "4 Cognitive Stages for Child Development." Accessed January 28, 2020. https://www.learningrx.com/4-cognitive-stages-for-child-development/.

Leitch, Carmen. "Remarkable Results from First Gene Therapy for Glycogen Storage Disease." Labroots. https://www.labroots.com/trending/genetics-and-genomics/15701/remarkable-results-gene-therapy-glycogen-storage-disease.

Mayo Clinic. "Liver Biopsy." November 24, 2020. https://www.mayoclinic.org/tests-procedures/liverbiopsy/about/pac-20394576.

Mayo Clinic. "PKU." Last modified May 13, 2022. https://www.mayoclinic.org/diseases-conditions/phenylketonuria/symptoms-causes/syc-20376302#:~:text=Phenylketonuria%20(fen%2Dul%2Dkey,needed%20to%20break%20down%20phenylalanine.

Moyer, Nancy. "Mast Cell Activation Syndrome." Healthline. Last modified July 13, 2022. Accessed May 13, 2020. https://www.healthline.com/health/mast-cell-activation-syndrome.

National Health Council. "About Chronic Diseases." July 29, 2014. Accessed February 25, 2020. https://nationalhealthcouncil.org/wp-content/uploads/2019/12/AboutChronicDisease.pdf.

Only the Bible. "Footprints in the Sand." Accessed January 20, 2020. https://www.onlythebible.com/Poems/Footprints-in-the-Sand-Poem.html.

Rajas, Fabienne, Julie Clar, Amandine Gautier-Stein, and Gilles Mithieux. "Lessons from New Mouse Models of Glycogen Storage Disease Type 1a in Relation to the Time Course and Organ Specificity of the Disease." *Journal of Inherited Metabolic Disease* 38, no. 3 (May 2015): 521–527. https://doi.org/10.1007/s10545-014-9761-0.

Rare Disease Database. "Glycogen Storage Disease Type I." NORD. Accessed January 22, 2020. https://rarediseases.org/rare-diseases/glycogen-storage-disease-type-i/.

Ross, Katalin. "General Nutrition Guidelines for Glycogen Storage Disease Type 1." Glycogen Storage Disease Program, University of Florida. 2008. Accessed January 30, 2020. https://ufhealth.org/sites/default/files/media/GSD/General-Nutrition-Guidelines-for-Glycogen-Storage-Disease-Type-I.pdf.

Ruddiman, Kathleen R., and Catherine Anastasopoulou. "Type 1a Glycogen Storage Disease Treatment and Management." Medscape. July 7, 2021. Accessed September 28, 2018. emedicine.medscape.com/article/119318-treatment#d8.

Shieh, Jeng-Jer, Mugen Terzioglu, Hisayuki Hiraiwa, Julia Marsh, Chi-Jiunn Pan, Li-Yuan Chen, Janice Yang Chou. "The Molecular Basis of Glycogen Storage Disease Type 1a." *Journal of Biological Chemistry* 277, no. 7. (February 2002): 5047-5053. Accessed September 28, 2018. https://doi.org/10.1074/jbc.M110486200.

Stevenson, Mary. "Footprints in the Sand." Footprints in the Sand. Accessed August 11, 2022. https://footprintssandpoem.com/mary-stevenson-version-of-footprints-in-the-sand/.

Storch, Eric, and Mary Keeley, Lisa Merlo, Marni Jacob, Catherine Correia, and David Weinstein. "Psychosocial Functioning in Youth with Glycogen Storage Disease Type 1." *Journal of Pediatric Psychology* 33, no. 7 (February 23, 2008): 728-38. Accessed September 23, 2019. https://doi.org/10.1093/jpepsy/jsn017.

Tolbert, Jennifer, Kendal Orgera, and Anthony Damico. "Key Facts about the Uninsured Population." KFF (November 6, 2020). https://www.kff.org/uninsured/issue-brief/key-facts-about-the-uninsured-population.

Ultragenyx. "DTX401: AAV8 Gene Therapy for Glycogen Storage Disease Type Ia (GSDla)." Accessed May 20, 2020. https://www.ultragenyx.com/pipeline/dtx-401-for-gsd1a/.

Ultragenyx. "Ultragenyx Announces First Patient Dosed in Phase 1/2 study of DTX401, a Gene Therapy for the Treatment of Glycogen Storage Disease Type Ia (GSDIa); FDA Grants Fast Track Designation to Gene Therapy Program." Globe Newswire. Accessed October 9, 2018. https://www.globenewswire.com/news-release/2018/07/26/1542689/0/en/Ultragenyx-Announces-First-Patient-Dosed-in-Phase-1

-2-study-of-DTX401-a-Gene-Therapy-for-the-Treatment-of-Glycogen-Storage-Disease-Type-Ia-GSDIa-FDA-Grants-Fast-Track-Designation-t.html.

University of Florida Health. "Gene Therapy." https://ufhealth.org/diabetes-center-excellence/research.

Walker, Jennifer. "Ground-Breaking Clinical Trial Participant First in the World to Receive Phase III Infusion for GSD Type 1a." *UConn Today*. January 20, 2022. https://today.uconn.edu/2022/01/ground-breaking-clinical-trial-participant-first-in-the-world-to-receive-phase-iii-gene-therapy-for-gsd-type-ia/.

Webb, Nancy Boyd, ed. *Helping Children and Adolescents with Chronic and Serious Medical Conditions*. Hoboken, NJ: Wiley and Sons, 2009.

Weinstock, Leonard B. "Approach to MCAS." Adapted from articles by Dr. Molderings and Dr. Afrin. Accessed May 20, 2020. http://www.gidoctor.net/client_files/File/Approach-to-MCAS-Dx-and-Rx-2-19.pdf (page discontinued).

Whelan, Corey. "Lactic Acidosis: What You Need to Know." Healthline. Last modified March 16, 2022. Accessed January 20, 2020. https://www.healthline.com/health/lactic-acidosis.

Wilson, SuLauren, "What Is a Feeding Tube, and How Do I Get Insurance to Pay for One?" Finnegan Medical Supply. September 2, 2014. https://finneganmedicalsupply.com/blogs/news/what-is-a-feeding-tube-and-how-do-i-get-insurance-to-pay-for-one.

Woods, Lauren. "World's Top Researcher of Rare Genetic Liver Disease Coming to Conn Health." UConn Today. September 19, 2016. Accessed November 1, 2018. https://today.uconn.edu/2016/09/worlds-top-glycogen-storage-disease-program-coming-uconn-health/.

ABOUT THE AUTHOR

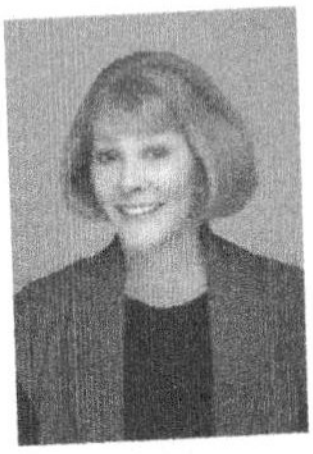

© DanielTurbert Photography

Janet Malcolm Hayles has been described as "very real, sometimes angry, sometimes tongue-in-cheek, and nearly always 'Kansan.'" A small-town, Kansas-born–turned–Jersey girl, Janet isn't afraid to take on a challenge. She pursued a bachelor's and a master's in English in her home state and later completed an MBA and accounting classes at Rockhurst University. Most recently, she received a master's in Graduate Liberal Studies from Duke University. Janet's varied career has ranged from writing humorous vignettes for various newspapers and magazines to spending nearly two decades in finance, accounting, and benefits to leading numerous speaking engagements. Her audiences have centered primarily the corporate world, for which she uses her voice to train individuals on effective communication and team building. Currently, she serves on the board of directors of her community's Property Owner's Association as well as the Learning Trail, an organization dedicated to tutoring Latinx children. She also writes and posts on her blog called *A Smile Every Monday* and contributes to her local periodicals.

Finally settled in North Carolina, Janet spends her days with her husband and new bichon puppy, Jean Claude, whose name is longer than he is (you can guess who has the real power in the house).

Made in United States
Orlando, FL
23 May 2023

33391670R00168